T0292264

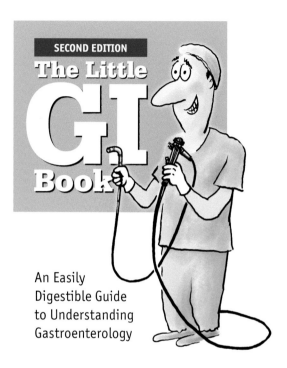

SECOND EDITION

The Little GI Book

An Easily
Digestible Guide
to Understanding
Gastroenterology

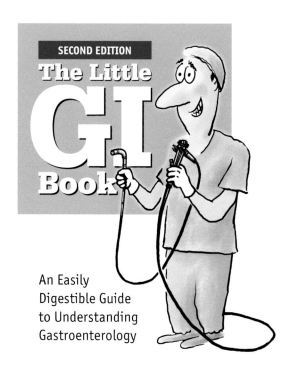

SECOND EDITION

The Little GI Book

An Easily
Digestible Guide
to Understanding
Gastroenterology

Douglas G. Adler, MD, FACG, AGAF, FASGE
Professor of Medicine
University of Utah School of Medicine
Salt Lake City, Utah

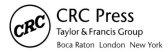

CRC Press
Taylor & Francis Group
Boca Raton London New York

CRC Press is an imprint of the
Taylor & Francis Group, an **informa** business

Illustrations done by Jeff Moore.

Dr. Douglas G. Adler is a consultant for Merit, BSC, Cook, Olympus, and Abbvie.

First published 2020 by SLACK Incorporated

Published 2024 by CRC Press
2385 NW Executive Center Drive, Suite 320, Boca Raton FL 33431

and by CRC Press
4 Park Square, Milton Park, Abingdon, Oxon, OX14 4RN

CRC Press is an imprint of Taylor & Francis Group, LLC

© 2020 Taylor & Francis Group, LLC

This book contains information obtained from authentic and highly regarded sources. While all reasonable efforts have been made to publish reliable data and information, neither the author[s] nor the publisher can accept any legal responsibility or liability for any errors or omissions that may be made. The publishers wish to make clear that any views or opinions expressed in this book by individual editors, authors or contributors are personal to them and do not necessarily reflect the views/opinions of the publishers. The information or guidance contained in this book is intended for use by medical, scientific or health-care professionals and is provided strictly as a supplement to the medical or other professional's own judgement, their knowledge of the patient's medical history, relevant manufacturer's instructions and the appropriate best practice guidelines. Because of the rapid advances in medical science, any information or advice on dosages, procedures or diagnoses should be independently verified. The reader is strongly urged to consult the relevant national drug formulary and the drug companies' and device or material manufacturers' printed instructions, and their websites, before administering or utilizing any of the drugs, devices or materials mentioned in this book. This book does not indicate whether a particular treatment is appropriate or suitable for a particular individual. Ultimately it is the sole responsibility of the medical professional to make his or her own professional judgements, so as to advise and treat patients appropriately. The authors and publishers have also attempted to trace the copyright holders of all material reproduced in this publication and apologize to copyright holders if permission to publish in this form has not been obtained. If any copyright material has not been acknowledged please write and let us know so we may rectify in any future reprint.

Library of Congress Cataloging-in-Publication Data
Names: Adler, Douglas G., 1969- author.
Title: The little GI book : an easily digestible guide to understanding
    gastroenterology / Douglas G. Adler.
Description: Second edition. | Thorofare, NJ : SLACK Incorporated, [2020] |
    Includes bibliographical references and index.
Identifiers: LCCN 2019051137 (print) | ISBN 9781630917418 (paperback)
Subjects: MESH: Gastrointestinal Diseases--therapy | Gastrointestinal
    Diseases--diagnosis
Classification: LCC RC801 (print) | NLM WI 140 | DDC
    616.3/3--dc23
LC record available at https://lccn.loc.gov/2019051137

ISBN: 9781630917418 (pbk)
ISBN: 9781003524885 (ebk)

DOI: 10.1201/9781003524885

DEDICATION

For my mother, and all that she does.

Contents

Dedication . . . . *v*
About the Author. . . . . *ix*
Preface . . . . *xi*
Preface to the First Edition . . . . *xiii*

Chapter 1   Esophagus 1
Chapter 2   Stomach 37
Chapter 3   Small Intestine. 71
Chapter 4   Colon and Rectum 99
Chapter 5   Liver 127
Chapter 6   Gallbladder and Bile Ducts 161
Chapter 7   Pancreas 193
Chapter 8   Endoscopy 225

Index. 273

ABOUT THE AUTHOR

Douglas G. Adler, MD, FACG, AGAF, FASGE attended SUNY Binghamton as an undergraduate and received his medical degree from Cornell University Medical College in New York, New York. He completed his residency in internal medicine at Beth Israel Deaconess Medical Center/Harvard Medical School in Boston, Massachusetts. Dr. Adler completed both a general gastrointestinal fellowship and a therapeutic endoscopy/endoscopic retrograde cholangiopancreatography (ERCP) fellowship at the Mayo Clinic in Rochester, Minnesota. He then returned to the Beth Israel Deaconess Medical Center for a fellowship in endoscopic ultrasound. Dr. Adler is currently a tenured Professor of Medicine and Director of Therapeutic Endoscopy at the University of Utah School of Medicine in Salt Lake City, Utah. Dr. Adler is also the GI Fellowship Program Director at the University of Utah School of Medicine. Working primarily at the University of Utah School of Medicine's Huntsman Cancer Institute, Dr. Adler focuses his clinical, educational, and research efforts on the diagnosis and management of patients with gastrointestinal cancers and complex gastrointestinal disease, with an emphasis on therapeutic endoscopy. He is the author of more than 400 scientific publications, magazine articles, and book chapters. This is Dr. Adler's eighth gastroenterology textbook.

PREFACE

The success of the first edition of this volume has been very gratifying to see. In my travels, I have met literally hundreds of students, nurses, physician assistants, and physicians who have told me that they had read *The Little GI Book* and how much it helped them learn the fundamentals of gastroenterology and hepatology.

In the years since *The Little GI Book* was published, much has changed in the world of gastroenterology and hepatology. This can be seen both with regard to diagnosis and treatment of many gastrointestinal disorders. The following are just a few examples:

- Hepatitis C is, for all intents and purposes, curable at the time of this writing.
- The use and role of biologics and biosimilars to treat inflammatory bowel disease have exploded.
- The development of transluminal stents has given rise to a whole new class of endoscopic procedures that were previously unimaginable.
- Endoscopic submucosal techniques have allowed endoscopic submucosal dissection, peroral endoscopic myomectomy, and gastric peroral endoscopic myomectomy to become commonplace at many institutions.

Advances like these, and many others, spurred me to produce a second edition of *The Little GI Book*. As I have gone through each of the chapters, I have added information on new diseases, medications, and procedures. Many new images have been added for this edition. I have removed out-of-date material as well. In contrast to the first edition, all of the endoscopic images in this volume are now in color, which should make them even more useful.

As with the first edition, I wrote this book with the broadest readership possible in mind. I know that, for many readers, this will be the first book on gastroenterology and hepatology they ever read, so I want to keep the tone and tenor of the book as accessible as possible.

I hope that you find reading this book as enjoyable as I found writing it!

Douglas G. Adler, MD, FACG, AGAF, FASGE
Salt Lake City, Utah

Preface to the First Edition

Gastroenterology is an exciting and fascinating field. No, really, it is.

This statement may come as a shock to many people; most individuals don't think that their digestive tract is exciting in any way. In all honesty, they are correct (the blood and guts of blood and guts is not exactly party talk). Most of us who practice gastroenterology and related fields didn't go into this business for the glamour.

Nonetheless, I stand by my original statement. Modern gastroenterology has evolved from a diagnostic discipline into a field that allows its practitioners to perform some of the most innovative therapeutic interventions in all of medicine on a daily basis. Gastroenterology incorporates a tremendous range of benign and malignant illnesses, includes patients from very young children to older adults, involves many organs (as opposed to some specialties that just focus on one organ), and allows those who practice it to treat and cure many maladies from the common to the obscure. We get to see and do amazing things all the time in this profession.

As you begin your study of gastroenterology, you will quickly find that there are many new concepts and terms to be absorbed in a rapid manner. Most of this can sound like incomprehensible jibber-jabber. People will hurl all manner of medical and surgical jargon your way and assume that you understand exactly what they mean (when you may not understand them at all!). It can be overwhelming to try to wrap your brain around all of this, especially if you've never heard it before, and many questions will cross your mind. What's the difference between a subtotal colectomy and a total proctocolectomy? How are colon and rectal cancers different (or are they really not different at all?) How can you tell if a patient has cirrhosis? What do you do next if he or she does have cirrhosis? If the patient is jaundiced, should you order an ultrasound, a magnetic resonance imaging scan, or an ERCP (and what the heck is an ERCP, anyway?)?

This is not a 1000-page, hardcover textbook of gastroenterology. In this book, which you can easily toss into your backpack or carry in the pocket of your white coat, I have attempted to provide the reader with a sort of "field guide" to gastroenterology. You should feel free to dog-ear the corners of the pages and highlight key passages as you see fit. Using an organ-based approach, we start at the top (the esophagus) and work our way down through the entire gastrointestinal tract to the very end (the colon and rectum). Don't be fooled—despite the small size of this book, there's a lot of valuable information here. I've worked hard to emphasize key concepts across all of gastroenterology for you. The chapters are designed to be easy to read, giving you a straightforward and practical understanding of gastrointestinal anatomy, physiology, disease states, and treatment. I have also included a wide range of images and figures to reinforce many of the core concepts in the text.

I wrote this book for a wide audience—medical assistants, nursing students, nurses and nurse practitioners, physician assistants, medical students, residents in medicine and surgery, and anybody else who wants a solid foundation for learning about gastroenterology will benefit from this book.

I hope that it is the first of many gastroenterology books you delve into during your career.

Douglas G. Adler, MD, FACG, AGAF, FASGE
Salt Lake City, Utah

Chapter 1

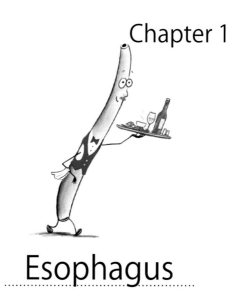

Esophagus

ANATOMY AND PHYSIOLOGY

Most people think the esophagus is simply a tube to carry food from the mouth to the stomach and never give it a second thought. In fact, the esophagus is a complex organ that performs a variety of functions, all of which we rely on to get us through each and every meal, drink, snack, and overindulgence.

The esophagus begins just below the upper esophageal sphincter, extends down through the chest, and ends at the level of the lower esophageal sphincter (LES), beyond which lies the stomach. Like all hollow gastrointestinal organs, the esophagus is composed of many layers and is not just a cylindrical piece of meat. The innermost lining

Adler DG. *The Little GI Book: An Easily Digestible Guide to Understanding Gastroenterology, Second Edition* (pp 1-36). © 2020 Taylor & Francis Group.

of the esophagus is referred to as the *mucosa*. Below the mucosa lies the submucosa and below that lies the muscularis propria, which allows the esophagus to contract. Beyond the muscularis propria lies the adventitia, which forms the outer coating of the organ.

The muscle in the esophagus is different at the top than it is at the bottom of the esophagus, and this is worth a few words of discussion. The muscle at the top is striated muscle, and the muscle at the bottom of the esophagus is smooth muscle. The muscle in the middle of the esophagus is somewhere between striated and smooth—a transition between the two. This is important because we can control striated muscle voluntarily, but we cannot control smooth muscle. What this really means is that we can initiate a swallow, but once the swallow starts, it proceeds automatically without conscious control. In other words, you cannot consciously stop a swallow once it is started.

When you are at rest, the esophageal sphincter, for the most part, stays closed (so that food and other unpleasant things do not come up out of your stomach and into your mouth), and the esophagus does not contract. Between meals, you swallow saliva from time to time. Occasionally, the sphincters will have brief episodes of relaxation, and this is important for certain diseases like gastroesophageal reflux disease (GERD), which we will cover a little later.

During a normal, healthy swallow, the upper esophageal sphincter relaxes, and food moves into the top of the esophagus (propelled by the tongue and the pharynx). The esophageal muscles contract in a coordinated and stepwise manner to push the food down through the esophagus toward the stomach. When the food gets to the bottom of the esophagus, the LES relaxes on schedule, and the food passes through into the stomach, where digestion can begin. Most of us swallow hundreds of times a day and never give it a second thought; the system works extremely well most of the time. When the system does not work well (ie, if the esophagus is diseased or there is a problem swallowing), people tend to notice it immediately. As a general rule, people with swallowing problems are said to have dysphagia.

DYSPHAGIA

Dysphagia can be caused by mechanical problems (eg, a tumor blocking the esophagus stricture, scar tissue), motility problems (ie, something is either wrong with the way the esophagus is contracting or with how the sphincters are functioning, and food is not being moved forward the way it should), or a combination of both.

Mechanical problems are, as a rule, easy to identify, although they may not be easy to treat. People with mechanical problems as a cause of their dysphagia tend to have more difficulty swallowing solids as opposed to liquids. This is because a chunk of meat will most likely get stuck, but a sip of juice can get through a narrow or partially blocked esophagus. Most people with mechanical problems will present to a gastroenterologist for evaluation at some point because solid food dysphagia is a very concerning symptom. Some of the most common mechanical problems that lead to dysphagia include esophageal cancer (which can occur anywhere in the esophagus), rings that can narrow the esophageal lumen (often referred to as *Schatzki rings*), webs (which can block the esophagus), scar tissue from prior surgery, and inflammatory strictures from GERD. Most benign strictures can be treated by dilation with a balloon or a dilation catheter (called a *bougie*). In some cases, the esophagus itself may be completely normal, but it is being compressed by an abnormal structure that is just next to it, such as a tumor in the lungs (imagine a foot stepping on a garden hose—there is nothing wrong with the hose itself except for the foot that is squashing it). Sometimes people have pockets in their esophageal walls that can trap food and make it hard to swallow. These pockets are usually referred to as *diverticula*.

In contrast, motility problems usually result in people having trouble swallowing both solids and liquids. In some patients with motility troubles, the esophagus looks normal when viewed via endoscopy but just does not work (contract) properly. Sometimes the problem can be with esophageal peristalsis, other times the sphincters do not work right, and sometimes both peristalsis and sphincter function are impaired. The upshot is that you need both a working esophagus and working sphincters to have a normal swallow.

Achalasia

The classic esophageal motility problem and the one you are most likely to be asked questions about is known as *achalasia*. Achalasia combines an LES that does not relax (even during a swallow when there is food in the esophagus) with a noncontractile, aperistaltic esophagus. This is really a double whammy—when people with achalasia swallow, the food goes into an esophagus that cannot contract and move it forward properly. When the food finally gets down to the distal esophagus, the sphincter does not relax to let the food into the stomach. People with achalasia have severe swallowing difficulties; they trap food in their esophagus where it goes bad (and smells terrible) and are at high risk for developing a type of esophageal cancer known as *squamous cell cancer* as a consequence of the disease. The exact cause of achalasia is unclear, but in some cases, it may be related to a type of parasitic infection known as Chagas disease (from the parasite *Trypanosoma cruzi*). Treatments for achalasia include a surgical myotomy (to physically cut the LES muscle so that it can stay open) performed with or without a fundoplication (where the top of the stomach is wrapped around itself to prevent acid reflux), injection of the neurotoxin/acetylcholine blocker known as *botulinum toxin* (Botox) into the LES (again so that it stays open), or dilation of the LES with very large balloons to stretch and partially tear muscle fibers in the LES (so that it stays open) so that food can get into the stomach.

A new treatment for achalasia that is rapidly becoming popular is known as a *peroral endoscopic myotomy* (POEM). In a POEM procedure, an endoscopist creates a submucosal tunnel in the esophagus that allows access to and direct visualization of the LES. This allows the endoscopist to cut the muscle directly, saving the patient from undergoing a surgery to perform this maneuver. POEM is still performed in a limited number of centers, but this is becoming more widely available.

Eosinophilic Esophagitis

Another common motility problem that you may encounter is referred to as *eosinophilic esophagitis*. Eosinophilic esophagitis is a very common cause of dysphagia and is often seen in young people. People with eosinophilic esophagitis have an esophagus that looks normal or may have a ringed appearance (like a cat's esophagus). These patients may have an esophagus with deep furrows or white plaques on the surface as well (Figure 1-1). When biopsied, the esophagus of a patient with eosinophilic esophagitis is rich in a kind of white blood cell called *eosinophils* (which often mediate allergic reactions). Patients with eosinophilic esophagitis often have a history of asthma, eczema, food allergies, and related problems. Eosinophilic esophagitis may also be related to acid reflux. Treatments for eosinophilic esophagitis usually include acid blockers (proton pump inhibitors [PPIs]), swallowed steroids, or other medications to decrease the number of eosinophils in the

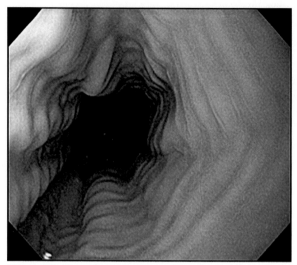

Figure 1-1. An endoscopic image of a patient with dysphagia and eosinophilic esophagitis. Note the ringed appearance of the esophagus, the linear furrows, and the narrowed lumen.

esophageal wall. Most patients respond well to medical therapy. You should think about eosinophilic esophagitis if you see a young person coming to the hospital for a food impaction (food, usually meat, stuck in his or her throat that has to be removed with an endoscope). These patients often have a narrow caliber esophagus that is prone to trapping foods and can be easily traumatized with an endoscope during endoscopy.

Other Esophageal Motility Disorders

Other esophageal motility problems that cause dysphagia include scleroderma (also sometimes referred to as *progressive systemic sclerosis*), where patients have poor esophageal contractility combined with an LES that stays open all the time and they develop chronic acid reflux that scars the esophagus, and spastic disorders of the esophagus, such as diffuse esophageal spasm and/or nutcracker esophagus. These last 2 disorders can produce severe pain as well as dysphagia. These diseases are often treated with PPIs, nitrates, and calcium channel blockers, but it can be very difficult to control these symptoms.

GASTROESOPHAGEAL REFLUX DISEASE

Pathophysiology

GERD represents one of the most common indications for a patient to be evaluated by a gastroenterologist. If you are reading this as a young person and have never experienced reflux or heartburn symptoms, you may wonder why there are so many television commercials for antireflux medications. If you are reading this and you are over 30 years old, you have very likely experienced reflux and/or heartburn at least once and know that the pain from this condition can be severe, can be extremely uncomfortable, and can last for hours at a time.

GERD is somewhat difficult to define, but a definition that most would agree on involves the reflux of gastric contents (that includes stomach acids as well as other substances, such as bile from the intestines and/or food) into the esophagus with the production of associated reflux symptoms, such as chest pain, heartburn, regurgitation, nausea, dysphagia, globus (a sensation of fullness in the neck), and water brash (hypersalivation), among others. Typical heartburn pain is retrosternal and is often severe. Patients may have difficulty concentrating, eating, or sleeping due to heartburn pain.

GERD can develop for a variety of reasons. Transient LES relaxations are thought to be the most common

mechanism causing GERD in patients with normal LES
resting pressures. Many patients also develop a hypotensive LES that serves as an inadequate barrier to keep
gastric contents out of the esophagus. A variety of conditions, foods, and medications can lead to a hypotensive
LES. Alcohol, caffeine, peppermint, and chocolate are
among the most common causes of a hypotensive LES. It
is often very difficult to convince patients to stop eating
these foods, even if they are having significant symptoms
of heartburn or reflux. (Would you want to stop eating
chocolate or drinking alcohol if a doctor told you to?)

Gastric distention, which is commonly seen after eating a large meal, is associated with a hypotensive LES
as well. The presence of a hiatal hernia, a condition in
which some of the acid-producing stomach slips through
the diaphragm and into the chest, is also a common etiology for a hypotensive LES. Obesity is also associated
with a hypotensive LES. Unfortunately, many patients
have a variety of potential etiologies simultaneously (ie, a
55-year-old obese woman with a large hiatal hernia who
drinks 4 cups of coffee per day is very likely to experience
heartburn symptoms).

Beyond being painful and uncomfortable, GERD is
a particular cause of concern because it is a commonly
recognized cause of a condition known as *Barrett's esophagus*. Barrett's esophagus involves the transition of the
normal squamous mucosal lining of the distal esophagus
into columnar cells (making the esophagus in some ways
mimic the appearance of the small bowel when viewed
under a microscope). Patients with Barrett's esophagus
are at increased risk of developing esophageal adenocarcinoma during their lifetime; thus, the presence of reflux
is directly related to the development of esophageal cancer in many patients. We will discuss Barrett's esophagus
in more detail a little later on.

It is worth noting that we do have some defenses
against GERD. Saliva contains significant amounts of the

alkali bicarbonate, which can help to neutralize gastric acid that makes it into the esophagus. A healthy LES prevents most acid and gastric contents from spilling back into the esophagus as well. In addition, an upright posture promotes the flow of any refluxed contents back down into the stomach. Thus, patients with decreased saliva production (smokers) are at increased risk for developing reflux, and many patients develop nocturnal reflux when lying flat in bed.

Diagnosis

Many patients will correctly diagnose themselves with esophageal reflux based on their symptoms. If a formal diagnosis of reflux (with or without esophagitis) is desired, this can be achieved via several means. The most common way that we diagnose patients with reflux is by directly visualizing an inflamed and/or ulcerated distal esophagus during an upper endoscopy (esophagogastroduodenoscopy). Reflux esophagitis can have a range of appearances that most gastroenterologists should be very comfortable identifying. These can include mild redness (erythema) in the distal esophagus, superficial ulcers, deep ulcers, frank bleeding, and acid-related esophageal strictures. Patients can have one or more of these features simultaneously. Some patients have a normal upper endoscopy in the setting of reflux or heartburn symptoms. These patients may have what is known as *nonerosive reflux disease.*

I should also point out that esophagitis can come from other causes besides GERD, so think of other possible etiologies when you see a patient with esophagitis. Fungal infections (usually from *Candida* species), viral infections (herpes simplex virus and cytomegalovirus), and medications (eg, bisphosphonates, tetracycline) can lead to esophagitis as well. Patients undergoing radiation therapy (for esophageal cancer, lung cancer, or other malignancies) can develop radiation esophagitis.

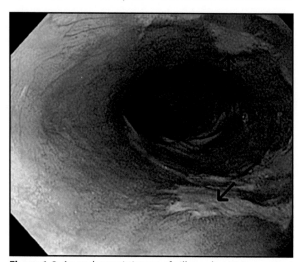

Figure 1-2. An endoscopic image of pill esophagitis in a patient taking tetracycline. There are focal "kissing" ulcers on opposite walls of the esophagus (arrows) from the edges of the pill itself.

Radiation esophagitis can be severe and can lead to chronic strictures of the esophagus that can be very difficult to treat. Pill esophagitis can occur when a medication in pill form that is itself caustic lodges in the esophagus and causes a direct chemical burn (Figure 1-2).

If endoscopy cannot be performed or is unrevealing and a diagnosis of reflux is still suspected, patients can undergo ambulatory esophageal pH monitoring. This can be performed using either a nasal esophageal catheter (which patients tend to dislike) or a wireless device that can be clipped into the distal esophagus (which is more comfortable but requires endoscopy to place). Both devices work equally well and can record the esophageal exposure to acid over a protracted period of time. In general, esophageal pH monitoring is performed for at least 24 hours, although sometimes longer studies are needed. It is of note that episodes of acid exposure may not directly correlate to symptoms of reflux or heartburn.

Esophageal manometry, which in the modern world is typically performed as high-resolution manometry, is a helpful test in patients in whom reflux (or dysphagia for that matter) is suspected to arise from an abnormal esophageal motility disorder. In this test, a catheter is placed into the esophagus that can measure upper and lower esophageal sphincter pressure as well as peristaltic contractions. Conditions associated with reflux, such as scleroderma, can easily be diagnosed via esophageal manometry. Other tests that can sometimes be used to diagnose acid reflux include the Bernstein test, which involves instilling acid into the patient's esophagus to see if it replicates his or her reflux symptoms (I promise I am not making that one up!), or an x-ray study in which the patient drinks contrast material and the radiologist looks to see if the contrast material flows back into the esophagus after it reaches the stomach. These last 2 tests are uncommonly used in the modern era.

Medical Treatment

Most patients with symptomatic acid reflux respond well to treatment. Before prescribing medications, it is always a good idea to see if the patient can respond to nonpharmacologic therapy in the form of lifestyle modifications. Some lifestyle modifications that we typically recommend patients try include stopping the consumption of trigger foods (eg, caffeine, chocolate) and/or alcohol (a relatively unpopular suggestion), losing weight, avoiding wearing tight clothing or tight pants, avoiding eating within several hours of going to sleep to allow the stomach to empty, chewing gum to promote salivation, stopping smoking, and elevating the head of the bed 6 to 8 inches to reduce nocturnal reflux events.

Although all of these lifestyle modifications are known to be highly effective in treating patients with symptomatic acid reflux, they are, in practice, poorly received by patients, and medical therapy is generally required. It is often extremely difficult to modify behaviors that may have been present for decades, and simply telling patients to change their lifestyle often has no effect on their actual behavior. Patients will often readily agree to change their lifestyle when confronted by an earnest physician wearing a white coat with a stethoscope around his or her neck, but the minute they return to their natural habitat, old habits generally resume.

Antacids

Antacids are the oldest and least expensive medications available to treat acid reflux. These drugs are inexpensive, available over the counter, and safe during pregnancy (for the most part); can help heal gastric and esophageal ulcers; and work well at preventing and controlling symptoms. Downsides to antacids include a relatively short duration of action and the need for frequent repeated doses.

H2 Receptor Antagonists

H_2 receptor antagonists (eg, cimetidine and ranitidine) represent a potent class of medications that block acid secretion from the gastric parietal cell by blocking H_2 histamine receptors. These agents are also available over the counter, are inexpensive, and are much more effective at treating symptoms and healing ulcers than simple antacids. These drugs are removed via hepatic and renal clearance and are relatively safe and well tolerated. Patients may develop tolerance to these drugs over time (known as *tachyphylaxis*) and may need drug holidays (a period of time where they have to stop taking the drug) to recover useful benefits from these agents.

Proton Pump Inhibitors

PPIs work by reversibly binding to the hydrogen-potassium ATPase found on the luminal surface of gastric parietal cells. Many PPIs are approved for use in the United States, including omeprazole/esomeprazole, lansoprazole/dexlansoprazole, rabeprazole, and pantoprazole. PPIs represent the most powerful antisecretory medications in widespread use around the world. Some PPIs are available via prescription only, and other PPIs are available over the counter. Most patients simply buy PPIs over the counter, and these are available as generic formulations, which helps patients to save money. PPIs cost more than other antisecretory agents, but patients do not develop tolerance to them, and they have a long duration of action (special long-acting PPIs are also available).

Other acid-blocking or antisecretory medications are available but are much less widely used than antacids, H2 blockers, and PPIs.

If the patient has typical symptoms in the presence of risk factors and the absence of alarm features in his or her history (bleeding, weight loss, and dysphagia), it is not unreasonable to simply try an empiric trial of medication in an attempt to reduce or relieve symptoms. In addition, many patients desire or require medications alongside lifestyle modifications to reduce their reflux symptoms. Some physicians like to try a step-up protocol to treat acid reflux (ie, start lifestyle modifications, begin antacids or H2 receptor blockers, and use PPIs as the last resort). Others like to go right to PPI therapy to get the patient the maximal symptomatic relief in the shortest time, albeit with the highest cost (this is known as a *top-down approach*). It is hard to say that one approach is better than the other, but if you experience reflux anytime soon, do not be surprised if you reach for a PPI before anything else because you are so miserable!

Other agents less commonly used to treat GERD include promotility agents, such as bethanechol and metoclopramide.

BARRETT'S ESOPHAGUS

Barrett's esophagus is an extremely common esophageal condition. It is hard for a gastroenterologist to go more than a few days without seeing a patient with Barrett's esophagus, and we talk about this disease all of the time.

A normal, healthy esophagus is lined by a flat squamous epithelium. In contrast, patients with Barrett's esophagus have a distal esophagus that is lined with a metaplastic columnar epithelium. This columnar epithelium has an atypical appearance that is usually easy to recognize endoscopically. The normal esophagus has a light, pale pink appearance, whereas Barrett's esophagus has a richer salmon-colored appearance. Barrett's esophagus also often has "tongues" of mucosa that can reach quite proximally in the esophagus.

Barrett's esophagus is a big deal. Why is a change in the lining of the esophagus such a big deal? Simply put, Barrett's esophagus is a precancerous condition. Patients with Barrett's esophagus are at an increased lifetime risk of developing esophageal adenocarcinoma, which is usually a fatal condition. These patients have about a 30-fold increased risk of developing esophageal adenocarcinoma during their lifetime (Figure 1-3). However, most patients with Barrett's esophagus will never develop esophageal cancer, but when looked at as a special subset of patients, their risk of cancer is quite high.

Diagnosis

In general, 2 things are required to diagnose a patient with Barrett's esophagus. First, an appearance suggestive

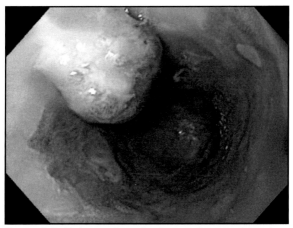

Figure 1-3. Early esophageal adenocarcinoma arising in a patient with Barrett's esophagus. Note the different appearance of the Barrett's mucosa in the distal esophagus.

of Barrett's esophagus (salmon pink distal esophagus) must be detected by endoscopy. Second, a biopsy must be obtained showing intestinal metaplasia (the formal term for the columnar cell-lined esophagus seen in Barrett's esophagus). The biopsy is critical for several reasons; it allows histologic confirmation of the presence of Barrett's esophagus, and it also allows evaluation for any dysplasia and the severity of that dysplasia. Dysplasia specifically refers to a precancerous change in the Barrett's esophagus itself. It is important to know if there is a dysplastic change in the Barrett's esophagus when deciding on management (either medical or surgical) and surveillance regimens. Most of the time, a gastroenterologist can be reasonably sure that he or she is seeing Barrett's esophagus simply based on the appearance of the esophagus, but we still biopsy anyway to be sure. Even experienced gastroenterologists can be wrong about the presence or absence of Barrett's esophagus based on appearance, and no matter how hard you try, you really cannot see dysplasia with a standard endoscope; you need a pathologist to tell you whether it is present or absent and to what level of severity. Most gastroenterologists perform 4 quadrant biopsies every 2 cm for the entire length of the Barrett's esophagus to adequately sample tissue.

Long- and Short-Segment Barrett's Esophagus

The squamocolumnar junction (known as the *Z line*) occurs at the bottom of the tubular esophagus. The gastroesophageal junction (GEJ) also occurs in the distal esophagus and marks where the esophagus ends and the proximal stomach begins. In a normal healthy patient, the squamocolumnar junction and the GEJ coincide (ie, the entire esophagus is lined by squamous epithelium). In patients with Barrett's esophagus, the squamocolumnar junction is proximal to the GEJ. If the squamocolumnar junction is less than 3 cm above the GEJ and the patient has Barrett's esophagus confirmed by biopsy, this is considered to be *short-segment* Barrett's esophagus. If the squamocolumnar junction is more than 3 cm above the GEJ in a patient with Barrett's esophagus confirmed on biopsy, this is considered to be *long-segment* Barrett's esophagus. This distinction is important. Patients with short-segment Barrett's esophagus may have less severe GERD or may have no GERD symptoms at all. Patients with long-segment Barrett's esophagus tend to have more severe GERD symptoms, including proximal esophageal acid exposure and nocturnal symptoms. Of greater importance, dysplasia and esophageal adenocarcinoma are much more common in patients with long-segment Barrett's esophagus when compared with short-segment Barrett's esophagus.

Prague Classification

When an endoscopist does an upper endoscopy on a patient with Barrett's esophagus, they often use the so-called *Prague classification* to describe what they see. The Prague classification uses 2 letters (C and M) and 2 numbers to describe a patient's Barrett's esophagus. The first landmark is taken from the beginning of the gastric folds, with 2 measurements being taken above this. The C refers to circumferential Barrett's and how high it extends from the gastric folds, and the M refers to the maximum proximal extent of the longest Barrett's segment. So, a patient with 2 cm of circumferential Barrett's mucosa and a tongue of mucosa that extends 5 cm from the gastric folds would be described as C2M5.

Management

The management of patients with Barrett's esophagus generally runs along 3 separate lines: surveillance, ablation or resection of the Barrett's mucosa, and acid suppression. Once the presence of Barrett's esophagus is established, all patients with the disease should undergo endoscopic surveillance with biopsies periodically. Most people use the guidelines on surveillance of Barrett's esophagus published by the American College of Gastroenterology. For patients with Barrett's esophagus and no dysplasia seen on 2 separate endoscopies within 1 year, follow-up endoscopy should be performed every 3 to 5 years, as long as no dysplasia is detected. Patients with low-grade dysplasia should be considered for endoscopic therapy to eradicate the Barrett's mucosa or could be considered to undergo periodic surveillance endoscopy as an alternative option if they cannot or do not want endoscopic therapy. Patients with high-grade dysplasia confirmed by an expert pathologist should undergo endoscopic therapy to eradicate the Barrett's mucosa. A rarely used option would be to undergo

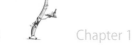

endoscopic treatment for the high-grade dysplasia in an attempt to eradicate it. Finally, if esophageal biopsies are indefinite for dysplasia, a repeat endoscopy after a trial of acid-suppressing medications (PPIs) should be performed. If the biopsy results on the second endoscopy confirm Barrett's esophagus that is indefinite for dysplasia, surveillance endoscopy with biopsies can be performed at 1 year.

Surgery

It is worth noting here that an esophagectomy is a major undertaking. An esophagectomy involves the removal of almost the entire esophagus and having the stomach pulled up vertically into the chest (where it is sewn into the very top of the remnant esophagus) to create a conduit for food to go from the mouth into the digestive system. An esophagectomy is one of the most complex, invasive, and unpleasant surgeries for a patient to undergo. Patients who are operated on by very experienced surgeons may still develop complications that can be severe, such as strictures at the site where the top of the esophagus is sewn onto the stomach. Many patients with Barrett's esophagus are elderly with other significant medical problems and may not be ideal candidates for surgery, especially major surgery. Given these facts, it might seem unlikely that anyone would choose esophagectomy in the setting of Barrett's esophagus with high-grade dysplasia, but in practice, some patients do select this option. People sometimes pick to undergo an esophagectomy because we know that high-grade dysplasia in a patient with Barrett's esophagus does not rule out the presence of a synchronous (ie, simultaneous) esophageal cancer, perhaps at a site in the Barrett's mucosa that was not sampled on recent biopsies. Our standard regimen of 4 quadrant biopsies every 2 cm per surveillance endoscopy is a good idea, but it is far from perfect, and if the patient is young and healthy enough

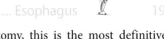

to undergo esophagectomy, this is the most definitive answer to avoid esophageal cancer.

Endoscopy

Endoscopic techniques to treat patients with Barrett's esophagus and high-grade dysplasia all use destructive methods to eliminate the Barrett's mucosa. The currently available endoscopic techniques involve the use of radio waves (radiofrequency ablation), heat (argon plasma coagulation), cold (cryotherapy), or destructive drugs that are activated by specific wavelengths of light delivered by a laser catheter (photodynamic therapy). Radiofrequency ablation is currently the most widely used technique. Radiofrequency ablation is currently the standard of care for patients with Barrett's esophagus and dysplasia (either low- or high-grade dysplasia) who want to have their Barrett's esophagus ablated. If patients have no dysplasia, radiofrequency ablation is not typically performed at most centers but can be done if the patient has worries about the risk of future cancer and is very motivated.

These approaches all work to varying extents, but each carries its own procedure-related risks, including the risk of inadequate treatment with the persistence of precancerous or frankly cancerous tissue in the Barrett's mucosa. If patients have nodules in the setting of their Barrett's esophagus, these are especially worrisome and are removed separately but with other endoscopic techniques such as endoscopic mucosal resection (EMR) and endoscopic submucosal dissection (ESD).

EMR has grown over the past few years into a widely used technique to remove growths on the lining of the gastrointestinal tract. EMR is an outgrowth of techniques developed to remove polyps in the colon and is now used in the esophagus, stomach, small bowel, and colon. EMR is very commonly used to remove nodular tissue arising in Barrett's esophagus that may harbor advanced precancerous tissue or even early-stage esophageal cancer. EMR involves the use of band ligators, very similar to those used to treat esophageal varices, to band abnormal tissue. The banding lifts the tissue up and makes it easier to remove, and the removal itself is usually done with an endoscopic snare and electrocautery. EMR used to be considered a high-end technique, but with the arrival of commercially available kits that contain all the devices one might need in a single box, EMR is now widely performed.

Closely related to EMR is ESD. ESD involves a more meticulous and aggressive dissection of abnormal growths lining the gastrointestinal tract and can be used to remove lesions that are too large to undergo EMR. Unlike EMR, ESD remains a high-end technique performed by a relatively small number of individuals. ESD can obviate surgery in many patients because lesions can be removed endoscopically. EMR and ESD are both used to remove early, superficial cancers of the esophagus. EMR and ESD come with risks such as perforation and bleeding, but they can be performed safely by experienced endoscopists.

Last, we always want to treat the underlying problem in patients with Barrett's esophagus and GERD. All patients with Barrett's esophagus should be placed on an aggressive antacid regimen of PPIs, almost always used in a twice-a-day formulation. The use of aggressive acid suppression probably has several benefits. First, it may promote the regression of Barrett's esophagus with restoration of the normal squamous epithelium. Second, it may slow or prevent the progression of Barrett's esophagus either in size (ie, the amount of esophagus involved) or in regard to the presence or severity of dysplasia. Third, it helps to control symptoms of GERD, which is very important to the patient. It may be worth considering a fundoplication as well because many patients with Barrett's esophagus have an underlying hiatal hernia, but this is not universally agreed on.

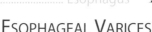

ESOPHAGEAL VARICES

Simply put, esophageal varices represent dilated esophageal veins that put patients at high risk of gastrointestinal bleeding. Patients with esophageal varices almost always have underlying portal hypertension, usually in the context of cirrhosis. Cirrhosis of any kind can lead to portal hypertension, and portal hypertension from any cause can lead to varices. We will cover esophageal varices in other chapters of this book as well, but it seems prudent to first discuss them here in the esophageal section so you can see them in the context of other diseases of the esophagus.

Pathophysiology

The portal vein is a large venous structure that runs through the liver. Patients with cirrhosis often develop outflow obstruction of the portal vein to varying degrees. When the pressure gradient between the portal vein and the hepatic veins gets too high (usually greater than 12 mm Hg), backflow in the venous system causes veins in the esophageal wall, which are usually collapsed, to distend with blood. These distended veins are then referred to as *varices*. Because these veins are not typically supposed to have flow in them and because patients with underlying liver disease often have a tendency toward bleeding, it is very common for these patients to develop variceal hemorrhage at some point in their lives. All patients with cirrhosis are typically screened periodically for esophageal varices, and those who are found to have them undergo treatment to try to eradicate the varices before they can bleed. If a patient develops a variceal bleed and was not known to have varices before this event, the varices can still be treated by a variety of methods. Variceal hemorrhage is often sudden in onset as well as severe and life- threatening, so a great deal of energy is put into avoiding variceal bleeds when at all possible.

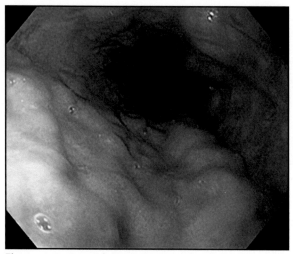

Figure 1-4. An endoscopic image of esophageal varices bulging into the esophageal lumen.

Endoscopic Evaluation

Most patients with known or suspected cirrhosis undergo periodic endoscopic evaluation to look for the presence or absence of varices (Figure 1-4). If varices are present, the gastroenterologist will evaluate them for their size (larger varices are more likely to bleed than smaller varices) and for other signs that suggest the varices are at high risk for bleeding. High-risk signs that can be seen during an endoscopic examination include the red wale sign (red lines on the surface of the varices), red spots, signs of recent hemorrhage like fresh or old blood in the esophagus, fibrin plugs on the varices, and tortuosity to the overall shape of the esophageal varices. Varices that flatten with air insufflation into the esophagus are at lower risk for bleeding than varices that do not collapse.

It is also important to take into account things such as the severity of the underlying cirrhosis, any history of variceal bleeding, and other factors when deciding how likely a patient is to experience a variceal bleed in the future.

Primary Prevention of Esophageal Variceal Bleeding Using Medications

If the patient is found to have esophageal varices and is at risk for variceal hemorrhage, steps to avoid the occurrence of a gastrointestinal bleed are warranted. The first line of treatment to prevent a first episode of variceal bleeding in patients with portal hypertension is the use of nonselective beta-blockers. These agents work by decreasing portal venous flow and can help decompress esophageal varices. Several nonselective beta-blockers are currently available in the United States, with propranolol and nadolol being the 2 most commonly used. These drugs can cause a significant reduction in the risk of a first episode of esophageal variceal bleeding. These drugs also decrease the patient's heart rate and are typically titrated to the point where the patient's heart rate is between 55 and 60 beats per minute. Giving more drugs above this level may result in the patient developing an unacceptably low heart rate, which can lead to other complications, such as episodes of syncope (fainting). Other agents are used as primary prevention of esophageal variceal bleeding (either alone or in combination with other drugs), but none are as widely used as the nonselective beta-blockers.

Endoscopic Therapy

Several endoscopic techniques are used to treat esophageal varices. These techniques can be used as primary prevention (in patients who have never bled) or as a secondary treatment (in patients who have recently bled or who are actively bleeding).

Band Ligation

Endoscopic band ligation represents the most widely used technique to treat esophageal varices in any situation. The technique is remarkably simple; a cap is fitted to the end of the endoscope, and the endoscope is advanced into the esophagus. When varices are identified, they are sucked into the cap on the tip of the endoscope, and what is essentially a very small and very strong rubber band is deployed around the varix. This rubber band cuts off all blood flow in the varix and also produces inflammation and thrombosis. Once banded, the varix itself will typically scar down, and the band will slough off at a later date. In contrast to early band ligators, which could only deploy one band at a time, modern endoscopic band ligators can deploy multiple bands without having to be removed from the patient. It is not uncommon to deploy 5 to 10 bands in a single procedure in a patient with multiple esophageal variceal trunks, often using multiple bands on the same variceal trunk at different distances from the incisors (Figure 1-5).

Endoscopic band ligation can be used in patients who have never bled (but who have high-risk stigmata as described previously) as well as patients with a history of past or active bleeding; the technique used is exactly the same. Once patients have had bands deployed, they generally need periodic re-examination to ensure complete eradication of all their esophageal varices. Patients who have had multiple episodes of banding of their varices often have an esophagus full of stellate scars, each one showing the location of a previously deployed band.

As fair warning to the reader, I should probably let you know that esophageal variceal banding can be quite painful for the patient. It is not uncommon to see patients grimacing and rubbing their hand over their chest in the recovery room after the procedure. This is not really surprising given the nature of the procedure overall. Most patients who undergo esophageal variceal banding

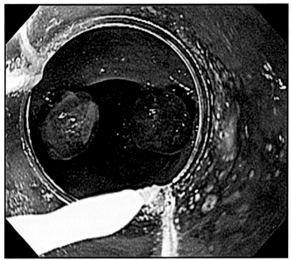

Figure 1-5. Two banded esophageal varices viewed endoscopically through a cap fitted to the end of an endoscope.

will request some sort of pain medication to control the pain. The pain usually lasts for several days and then fades away. After esophageal banding is performed, it is generally a good idea to place patients on a liquid diet for 1 or 2 days because their swallowing may be impaired by the presence of all the banded varices in the esophagus. Once in a blue moon, you will read or hear about a patient who developed esophageal obstruction after banding of esophageal varices, but this is a very rare event.

Sclerotherapy

Another treatment for esophageal varices you should be aware of is known as *sclerotherapy*. Sclerotherapy involves injecting sclerosing agents into the varices to promote inflammation and clot formation as well as scarring. A variety of sclerosing agents are commercially available. For many years, sclerotherapy was the gold standard approach to the endoscopic treatment of esophageal varices, but, given the rise of endoscopic band ligation over the past 25 years, sclerotherapy is much less commonly used. Most physicians use sclerotherapy when endoscopic band ligation has been attempted and is unsuccessful in treating a patient with active variceal bleeding. The sclerosing agents used in sclerotherapy are also quite toxic and have to be handled with extreme care. Exposure of these agents to the eye, for example, can result in serious injury.

Shunts and Balloons

If endoscopic therapy with bands or sclerotherapy fails to treat a patient with active variceal hemorrhage, other techniques can be used in an attempt to save the patient's life, such as the creation of a decompressing portosystemic shunt (which is performed by interventional radiologists and not gastroenterologists). This shunt may be referred to as a *transjugular intrahepatic portosystemic shunt*. Another option is the use of an esophageal balloon to compress and tamponade the varices (known as a *Blakemore tube* or a *Sengstaken-Blakemore tube* if there is an additional balloon to compress gastric varices). Patients who do not have their bleeding stopped by endoscopic approaches and need either a transjugular intrahepatic portosystemic shunt or an esophageal balloon are at very high risk of dying.

ESOPHAGEAL CANCER

The term *esophageal cancer* refers to tumors of the esophagus that arise from its most superficial lining, the mucosa. The overwhelming majority of esophageal cancers are either squamous cell cancers or adenocarcinomas.

Historically, squamous cell cancers were very commonly seen, and adenocarcinomas were rare entities. This trend has reversed over the past several decades, with a significant rise in the incidence of esophageal adenocarcinoma. Currently, esophageal adenocarcinomas outnumber squamous cell carcinomas. Esophageal squamous cell cancers typically develop in the upper and middle portions of the esophagus, whereas adenocarcinomas almost always involve the distal esophagus. Tumors that involve the distal esophagus and the proximal stomach are often referred to as *junctional tumors* because they span the esophagogastric junction. These tumors are also virtually always adenocarcinomas.

Etiology

The main risk factors for esophageal squamous cell cancer include tobacco use, alcohol consumption, prior head and neck cancer, lye ingestion, and achalasia. Lye, typically found in over-the-counter household cleaning products, is often ingested during suicide attempts. Lye ingestion typically leads to severe inflammation and stricture formation in the esophagus and can give rise to squamous cell cancer many years later.

The number one risk factor for the development of esophageal adenocarcinoma is Barrett's esophagus. GERD is commonly associated with Barrett's esophagus, as we discussed previously, and GERD itself is independently linked to the development of esophageal adenocarcinoma. Obesity is also an independent risk factor for esophageal adenocarcinoma, probably because obese patients are at increased risk for GERD and, in turn, Barrett's esophagus.

A prior history of esophageal cancer is also a risk factor for the future development of esophageal cancer. Patients who undergo an esophagectomy can still develop recurrent esophageal cancer, most notably adenocarcinoma.

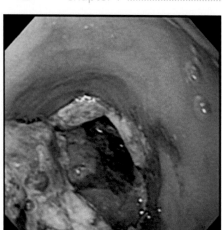

Figure 1-6. An obstructing esophageal cancer causing malignant dysphagia.

Clinical Presentation and Pretreatment Evaluation

A few lucky patients have their esophageal cancers discovered incidentally during upper endoscopy either for unrelated causes or during the surveillance of Barrett's esophagus. Patients with early-stage esophageal cancer can often undergo endoscopic removal of the tumor or an esophagectomy with a very high chance of complete curative resection.

Unfortunately, most patients with esophageal cancer present with relatively advanced disease (Figure 1-6). The reason that most patients present with late-stage disease is that most early tumors are asymptomatic. Surprisingly, patients can have a relatively large esophageal lesion and still not develop dysphagia (hence the common delay in the diagnosis of these cancers). The presence of dysphagia to solid foods, weight loss, episodes of food impaction, and other alarming features typically drives patients to see their physicians, which ultimately leads to some sort of imaging study or endoscopy that discloses the presence of the tumor. Historically, esophageal cancers were typically diagnosed via barium swallow or other radiographic studies, but currently the overwhelming majority of esophageal cancers are diagnosed during an upper endoscopy in which a biopsy is obtained.

Once a patient has been diagnosed with esophageal cancer of any type, the next best test to obtain is a computed tomography (CT) scan of the chest, abdomen, and pelvis to look for the spread of the tumor to other organs. These satellite tumors are referred to as *metastases*. If the CT scan discloses metastatic disease, the patient has stage IV disease, and his or her disease is unresectable and, for all intents and purposes, incurable.

If the patient does not have evidence of spread to other organs on CT scanning, the patient should undergo an endoscopic ultrasound (EUS) examination. EUS refers to endoscopic examination with special endoscopes that not only have a light and a camera built into them but also an ultrasound transducer. EUS allows the endoscopist to not only see the tumor but also to see through the tumor and into the surrounding thoracic and abdominal structures (Figure 1-7). Regular endoscopes can only biopsy tissue that they can see directly. EUS scopes have the advantage of being able to biopsy tissue that cannot be seen endoscopically but rather only on ultrasound. EUS scopes have the capacity to perform fine-needle aspiration through the esophageal wall and into suspicious peritumoral lymph nodes to definitively assess for the presence or absence of cancer in those lymph nodes.

We discussed earlier that the esophageal wall is made up of many layers. Esophageal cancer staging is dependent on the assessment of what layers of the esophageal wall the tumor has invaded. Tumors that only invade

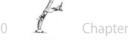

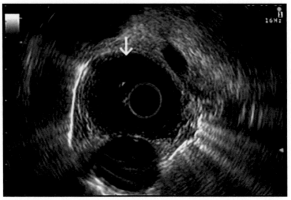

Figure 1-7. An EUS image of the same patient in Figure 1-6. The esophageal cancer has obliterated all esophageal wall layers. The tumor is the irregularly shaped dark lesion (arrow) surrounding the endoscope that lies at the center of the screen. The dark circle at the bottom of the image is the aorta.

the mucosa and submucosa are potentially removable by endoscopic techniques only, such as EMR. Tumors that are too big to be removed endoscopically but still only invade the mucosa and submucosa can be removed by proceeding directly to surgery in the form of esophagectomy. Tumors that invade the deeper layers of the esophagus, such as the muscularis propria or the adventitia, or tumors of any depth of invasion that have associated malignant lymph nodes require additional treatments before surgery, known as *neoadjuvant therapy*.

Neoadjuvant Therapy and Subsequent Esophagectomy

Neoadjuvant therapy typically consists of a combination of chemotherapy and radiation therapy delivered over the course of several months. Neoadjuvant therapy is administered to the patient by a medical oncologist

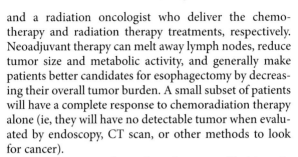

and a radiation oncologist who deliver the chemo-therapy and radiation therapy treatments, respectively. Neoadjuvant therapy can melt away lymph nodes, reduce tumor size and metabolic activity, and generally make patients better candidates for esophagectomy by decreasing their overall tumor burden. A small subset of patients will have a complete response to chemoradiation therapy alone (ie, they will have no detectable tumor when evaluated by endoscopy, CT scan, or other methods to look for cancer).

Many patients with esophageal cancer will ultimately proceed to esophagectomy if they do not have an early esophageal cancer that can be removed with an endo-scope. Esophagectomy should be performed by an experienced surgical oncologist, hopefully at a high-volume cancer center. As we mentioned earlier, the surgery is a major undertaking and is not without risks, even in the hands of an expert.

Endoscopic Treatments for Dysphagia in Esophageal Cancer

Most patients with esophageal cancer will develop dysphagia at some point during their disease. If the patient proceeds directly to surgery, usually no additional treatments for his or her dysphagia are needed because the tumor will simply be removed during the operation (unless he or she develops a postoperative stricture). If the patient has unresectable disease and a large tumor that causes dysphagia or has a potentially resectable tumor but must undergo neoadjuvant therapy before surgery first, treatment for dysphagia is usually desired. Treating a patient's dysphagia has several benefits—it allows patients to take nutrition and hydration by mouth, and it also allows patients to take medications by mouth. In addition, most patients simply feel better when they can eat and drink without the fear of food becoming stuck in their esophagus.

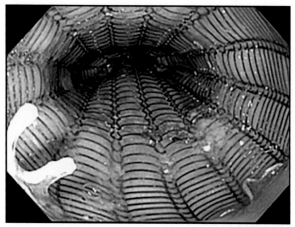

Figure 1-8. Image of esophageal stent placed to relieve obstruction in the same patient from Figure 1-6.

Stents

The most common treatment for dysphagia in patients with preoperative or nonoperative esophageal cancer is a self-expanding stent (Figure 1-8). These stents can either be made of metal or plastic and are inserted endoscopically. The stents are supplied from their manufacturers on thin delivery catheters, and when placed across the tumor and deployed in the esophagus, they shorten in terms of length and expand in terms of width. The stents hold the esophagus open and allow the patient to have improvement in his or her symptoms of dysphagia.

Esophageal stents are available in 2 varieties: fully covered or partially covered. Fully covered stents are constructed of a metal mesh or a plastic mesh coated with silicone or other thin plastic materials. Fully covered stents have the advantage of being potentially removable at some later date because their coating prevents them from permanently embedding into the surrounding esophageal wall. The drawback of these devices is that fully covered stents are more prone to migration because the coating reduces their ability to anchor their position in the esophagus. Partially coated stents (in which a portion of the metal mesh that makes up the stent is not coated and the bare wires of the stent are exposed) are generally used in patients with unresectable disease in whom there is no plan to ever remove the stent. It is very uncommon for a partially covered esophageal stent to migrate because tumor tissue can grow through the uncovered portion of the stent, helping to anchor them into position.

Self-expanding stents are widely used to treat dysphagia from esophageal cancer. These devices also have a role in the treatment of benign strictures of the esophagus, as well as a variety of other difficulties. Some patients with esophageal cancer (or lung cancers that invade the esophagus) can develop a hole between their airway and the esophagus, known as a *tracheoesophageal fistula* (TEF). A TEF can be a medical emergency because whenever the patient tries to swallow, he or she can pass swallowed solids or liquids into his or her lungs. This can lead to shortness of breath, pneumonia, and other severe difficulties. Esophageal stents are often used to cover up the TEF and allow patients to swallow safely. Esophageal stents can also be used to cover up holes in the esophagus that occur spontaneously (Boerhaave syndrome), from iatrogenic causes (endoscopy with perforation of the esophagus), or from trauma in selected patients.

Although stents can provide the patients with significant improvement in their level of dysphagia, it is important to remember that they are far from perfect devices. Esophageal stents typically do not allow patients to eat anything they want as soon as they are deployed. Unfortunately, you cannot go to an all-you-can-eat Las Vegas buffet with an esophageal stent in. This is not surprising because esophageal stents have no ability to produce peristaltic contractions like the normal esophagus does to help food move along and into the stomach. Most patients with an esophageal stent can return to a diet of soft foods and are usually able to drink any liquid without difficulty. Very few patients with an esophageal stent can eat a completely normal diet. In addition, the stents carry risks of complications, including pain, esophageal perforation, bleeding, and migration of the stent out of the esophagus and into the stomach (where it can no longer help treat the patient's dysphagia). Most patients tolerate stents well, but if complications arise, they can be serious.

Other Endoscopic Approaches to Treat Dysphagia in Esophageal Cancer

Other endoscopic treatments for dysphagia include ablative techniques such as laser therapy or argon plasma coagulation that simply burn away obstructing esophageal tumor tissue. Cryotherapy can be used to freeze tumor tissue and destroy it (Figure 1-9). If patients are not felt to be candidates for stenting or do not want an esophageal stent, they can have a feeding tube placed. Feeding tubes allow medications, nutrition, and hydration to be delivered to the patient's digestive system, but they do not allow a return to eating by mouth. Nasogastric tubes (that go from the nose through the esophagus and into the stomach), gastrostomy tubes (that go through the abdominal wall and into the stomach), and jejunostomy tubes (that go through the abdominal wall and directly into the small bowel) are all commonly used in esophageal cancer patients. The selection of a particular type of tube is often individualized depending on the patient's overall situation.

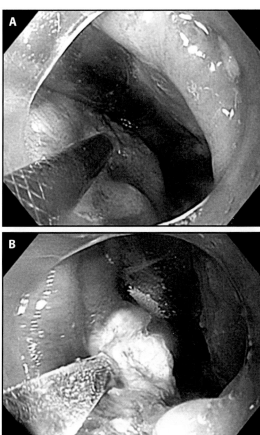

Figure 1-9. (A) An endoscopic image of an esophageal cancer that is to be treated with cryotherapy. Note the cryotherapy delivery catheter on the left side of the image, which will spray frozen liquid nitrogen directly onto the tumor. (B) The same patient as in Figure 1-9A. Cryotherapy is being applied, and the tumor is being frozen and can be seen to be covered with white frost.

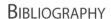

BIBLIOGRAPHY

Adler DG, Romero Y. Primary esophageal motility disorders. *Mayo Clin Proc*. 2001;76(2):195-200.

Almansa C, Devault KR, Achem SR. A comprehensive review of eosinophilic esophagitis in adults. *J Clin Gastroenterol*. 2011;45(8):658-664.

Brimhall B, Adler DG. Esophageal stents for the treatment of malignant dysphagia in patients with esophageal cancer. *Hosp Pract (1995)*. 2010;38(5):94-102.

Hu S, Adler DG. Endoscopic cryotherapy. Indications and efficacy. *Pract Gastroenterol*. 2015;22:19-45.

Patti MG, Pellegrini CA. Esophageal achalasia 2011: pneumatic dilatation or laparoscopic myotomy? *J Gastrointest Surg*. 2012;16(4):870-873.

Qureshi W, Adler DG, Davila R, et al; Standards of Practice Committee. ASGE Guideline: the role of endoscopy in the management of variceal hemorrhage, updated July 2005 [erratum in *Gastrointest Endosc*. 2006:63(1):198]. *Gastrointest Endosc*. 2005;62(5):651-655.

Schlottmann F, Patti MG. Laparoscopic Heller myotomy versus per oral endoscopic myotomy: evidence-based approach to the treatment of esophageal achalasia. *Am Surg*. 2018;84(4):496-500.

Siddiqui AA, Sarkar A, Beltz S, et al. Placement of fully covered self-expandable metal stents in patients with locally advanced esophageal cancer before neoadjuvant therapy. *Gastrointest Endosc*. 2012;76(1):44-51.

Chapter 2

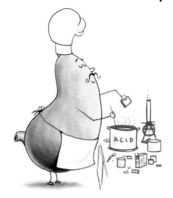

Stomach

Just as the esophagus is more than a tube, the stomach is more than just a place to put cheeseburgers and fries on a Friday night! The stomach serves many important functions in normal health and digestion. The stomach is also a common location for gastrointestinal disease to occur. This chapter will review the basics of gastric anatomy and physiology, as well as some of the most common disease states of the stomach that you will encounter in clinical practice.

Adler DG. *The Little GI Book: An Easily Digestible Guide to Understanding Gastroenterology, Second Edition* (pp 37-70).
© 2020 Taylor & Francis Group.

ANATOMY

The stomach is a hollow, muscular organ whose primary purpose is to be a repository for ingested food and a place for the process of digestion to begin. Like all of the hollow gastrointestinal organs, the wall of the stomach is made up of multiple layers of muscle and connective tissue that allow the stomach to contract in an accorded manner. The innermost layer of the gastric wall is known as the *mucosa*, and the mucosa contains a variety of cell types that allow for normal gastric acid secretion (more on this later).

The stomach sits between the esophagus and the small bowel. The stomach begins just below the gastroesophageal junction and terminates just beyond the pylorus, at which point the small bowel begins. The stomach is divided into several parts. It is sometimes difficult to say exactly where one portion of the stomach ends and another begins, but, as a general rule of thumb, endoscopists, surgeons, radiologists, and other health care providers generally agree on the following:

- The topmost portion of the stomach, located just below the lower esophageal sphincter, is referred to as the *gastric cardia*.
- The gastric fundus is the dome- or cap-like portion of the stomach that is usually underneath the left hemidiaphragm.
- The gastric body is the central portion of the stomach. The medial wall of the gastric body is referred to as the *lesser curvature*, whereas the lateral wall of the gastric body is referred to as the *greater curvature*.
- The distal most portion of the stomach is known as the *antrum*. The antrum terminates in the pylorus, which is the entry point into the small bowel

and the end of the stomach. The pylorus itself is surrounded by a strong muscular ring that helps food move into the small bowel for the next phase of digestion.

The stomach performs an interesting function known as *accommodation*. Accommodation refers to the fact that when you start to eat, your stomach will passively relax to allow your body to hold a large amount of food in one sitting. It is true that your stomach "shrinks" between meals, but this is really just the flip side of being able to expand greatly during mealtimes. The stomach is lined by thick folds known as *rugae*. The rugae are part of the secret of gastric accommodation; when the stomach collapses, the lining becomes thickly folded, and when the stomach needs to expand, the folds flatten out to create an increased surface area within the stomach itself. Gastric accommodation is what allows us to enjoy large meals, such as buffets in Las Vegas!

GASTRIC ACID PRODUCTION

Everybody knows that the stomach produces acid, but most people do not know how or, more importantly, why this is the case. From a clinical point of view, the production of acid by the stomach is vitally important to understand. Many common gastrointestinal disease states are directly related to gastric acid production.

The stomach does not just produce acid; the stomach produces something known as *gastric juice*. Gastric juice is predominantly made of hydrochloric acid. The hydrochloric acid is produced by cells known as *parietal cells*, which are found in the gastric mucosa. Gastric juice also contains mucus and electrolytes. Parietal cells can make acid in response to certain stimulating hormones and can stop making acid in response to certain inhibiting hormones. The substance histamine, the neurotransmitter acetylcholine, and the hormone gastrin all promote gastric acid secretion from parietal cells, whereas the hormone somatostatin and other chemicals known as *prostaglandins* can reduce parietal cell acid production and secretion. Gastrin is produced by cells known as *G cells*, whereas somatostatin is produced by cells known as *D cells*. Both G and D cells are found in the gastric mucosa. Histamine is produced by something known as an *enterochromaffin-like cell*, which, as you would expect by now, is also found in the gastric mucosa.

Why Does Your Stomach Produce All This Acid?

Most people think that the stomach produces acid so that the acid itself can break down food they eat; this is not really the case. The acid has 2 main functions. First, the acid helps sterilize the contents of the stomach in an attempt to kill any bacteria that you may have ingested as a means of preventing you from getting sick. People who take acid blockers are at increased risk of certain gastrointestinal infections because they are reducing the level of acid in their stomach. Second, the acid lowers the pH of the stomach to the point where a group of enzymes, known as *proteases*, can function. Proteases serve to break down ingested protein, and, thus, within the stomach, the digestion of protein begins. The process continues in the small bowel (along with many other digestive activities), but, again, protein digestion really starts in the stomach. These proteases, known as *pepsins*, are secreted into the stomach in protoforms known as *pepsinogens*. Pepsinogens are produced by chief cells and mucus cells that live in the gastric lining (mucosa). The protoforms of these proteases become active in the stomach when exposed to the low pH produced by the acid itself.

Why Doesn't This Acid Burn a Hole in Your Stomach?

You might wonder why all this acid does not result in your stomach burning all the time and why you do not develop holes in your own stomach as well. The truth is that some people *do* have gastric burning from too much acid, and some people *do* make holes in their stomach from too much acid! We will talk more about peptic ulcer disease in a little while, but the good news is that most patients will go their whole lives without having any gastric disorders due to acid. Your stomach contains a variety of defense mechanisms to protect itself from the acid that it produces. The mucus that the lining of your stomach produces helps insulate the cells that produce the acid from the acid itself. The mucus also contains secreted bicarbonate (HCO_3^-) that helps to neutralize the acid directly. In addition, the vigorous blood supply to the stomach helps to carry away any excess acid from the gastric mucosa.

VITAMIN B_{12}

Vitamin B_{12} metabolism is complex (most doctors have to look this up and refresh their memory on this topic every once in a while) but is worth some discussion because it is related to gastric physiology. Stomach acid and the enzyme pepsin cleave vitamin B_{12} from food particles, where it then binds to stabilizing proteins (known as *R proteins*, made via the salivary glands). Vitamin B_{12} is then severed from digested R proteins in the duodenum via pancreatic enzymes, where it can then bind to an agent known as *intrinsic factor* (IF), which is manufactured by parietal cells in the stomach. The IF/B_{12} complex then passes through the small bowel, where it is absorbed in the terminal ileum. Got it? Good!

The reason this is relevant to the stomach chapter of this book is that a common condition called *atrophic gastritis* often leads to vitamin B_{12} deficiency. Patients with atrophic gastritis may have antibodies to parietal cells and/or IF; thus, their vitamin B_{12} metabolism goes awry, and vitamin B_{12} deficiency develops.

HIATAL HERNIAS

Most people have heard of hiatal hernias but really have no idea what they are. People hear the term *hernia* and think of a problem around their belly button or maybe even in their groin. Hernias do occur at those locations, but hiatal hernias are actually hernias of the stomach itself. The term *hiatal hernia* refers to a portion of the stomach passing through the diaphragm and into the chest through the hole in the diaphragm (the diaphragmatic hiatus) that allows the esophagus to pass into the stomach. This can happen as a normal part of aging or when there is a tear or defect in the diaphragm.

Hiatal hernias can be small or large; some patients may only have a few centimeters of their stomach above the diaphragm, whereas other patients can have significant amounts of their stomach no longer contained within the abdominal cavity.

The vast majority of hiatal hernias are asymptomatic or produce only minimal symptoms, such as occasional heartburn or dyspepsia. Most patients with hiatal hernias have what are referred to as *sliding hiatal hernias*. These types of hiatal hernias involve a small amount of stomach slipping through the diaphragm and are referred to as *sliding* because the stomach periodically slips up into the chest and then back down into the normal position below the diaphragm in the abdomen.

Some hiatal hernias, known as *paraesophageal hernias*, involve a portion of the stomach slipping through the diaphragmatic hiatus next to the esophagus and pinching a portion of the stomach into the thorax.

Patients with hiatal hernias can have no symptoms or may have symptoms such as gastroesophageal reflux disease (GERD), the feeling of fullness in their chest, chest pain that may be severe enough to mimic a heart attack, or difficulty swallowing (dysphagia). Some patients can develop gastrointestinal bleeding from ulcers or erosions that form along the edge of the hernia due to mechanical trauma. These ulcers are known as *Cameron's erosions* (after Alan Cameron of the Mayo Clinic). Cameron's erosions generally do not improve with proton pump inhibitor therapy because they are not an acid-mediated phenomenon.

Risk Factors

A variety of situations put patients at risk for the development of a hiatal hernia. Some of these can be modified by the patient, whereas others the patient has no control over. It is also fair to say that some people develop hiatal hernias in the absence of any of the following risk factors:

- Age: Most patients with hiatal hernias are older than 40 years
- Weight gain and/or obesity
- Pregnancy
- Chronic and/or severe vomiting
- Chronic and/or severe coughing
- Straining during bowel movements (which raises intra-abdominal pressure)
- Heavy lifting

Treatment

If a hiatal hernia is small and the patient has minimal to no symptoms, no specific treatment may be indicated. If the hernia is large and/or the patient is symptomatic (most notably with GERD, chest pain, or dysphagia), then therapy should be considered. Therapeutic options include the following:

- Weight loss (easy to say, hard to do!)
- Use of acid-suppressing medications to control symptoms such as GERD
- Surgery
    - Several operations to treat symptomatic hiatal hernias are available, with the most common being Nissen fundoplication. This term refers to a procedure in which the hernia is reduced back into the abdomen below the diaphragm, and the fundus of the stomach is wrapped around the distal esophagus. In this manner, if all goes well, the stomach can no longer herniate through the diaphragm, and the patient's symptoms should resolve. Other surgical options allow the surgeon to make the opening from the esophagus into the stomach more or less tight as desired.

It should be noted that most patients with hiatal hernias never need surgery. The downsides to surgery include the fact that the stomach may "unwrap" itself, and the patient may return to his or her normal anatomy over time (often with recurrence of the hiatal hernia). If the wrap is made too tight, patients may have difficulties with swallowing or vomiting. Some patients also have trouble burping after undergoing fundoplication (a situation referred to with the unfortunate moniker of *gas-bloat syndrome*). Sometimes these symptoms can be treated by endoscopic balloon dilation of the distal esophagus/

proximal stomach, and sometimes they are so severe that the patient requires a second surgery to correct them.

PEPTIC ULCER DISEASE

Peptic ulcer disease represents one of the most commonly encountered clinical problems seen in gastroenterology. It is truly the bread and butter of gastroenterologists around the world. An enormous amount of time and energy during the training of gastroenterologists goes into learning how to evaluate and treat patients with known and suspected peptic ulcer disease.

The term *peptic ulcer disease* specifically refers to a breakdown of the lining of the stomach and/or the proximal duodenum with resulting ulcer formation and its attendant complications. Although these ulcers can occur in the duodenum as mentioned previously, peptic ulcer disease is largely thought of as a gastric problem due to the nature of how these ulcers form and are treated.

Peptic ulcer disease can arise in a variety of disease states, including the following:

- **Use of nonsteroidal anti-inflammatory drugs (NSAIDs):** NSAID use can, to a limited extent, cause direct mucosal injury to the stomach and the small bowel but, more commonly, can cause ulcers via the inhibition of cyclooxygenase 1 (COX-1). COX-1 is an enzyme that plays a key role in the protection of the gastrointestinal tract from the acidic environment of the stomach. This enzyme is responsible for the production of chemicals known as *prostaglandins*, which are in turn responsible for the production of mucus and bicarbonate by the gastric cell lining as well as the enhancement of blood flow, all of which serve as protective measures against gastric acid. NSAIDs reversibly inhibit COX-1, which can lead to the formation of ulcers via the loss of these protective mechanisms in a milieu of constant acid exposure. It should be noted that aspirin in particular irreversibly inhibits COX-1, making it even more ulcerogenic. The combination of corticosteroids and NSAIDs is particularly ulcerogenic.

- **Infection with *Helicobacter pylori*:** *H pylori* are gram-negative bacteria that are often found in the stomach and are a direct cause of peptic ulcer disease in a vast number of people worldwide. Although *H pylori* infection occurs in every country on the globe, it is more commonly seen in developing countries than in developed nations. *H pylori* infection can occur even in the acidic stomach because the organism produces an enzyme known as *urease*. Urease allows *H pylori* to cleave urea into carbon dioxide and ammonia. Ammonia is then used to buffer acid around the organism and create a more neutral pH environment. Infection with *H pylori* produces significant inflammation in the gastric wall, which, when combined with ongoing gastric acid and pepsin secretion, leads to a breakdown in the lining of the gastric wall and the formation of ulcers.

- **Stress ulcers:** Severe physiologic stress (not emotional stress!) can also lead to the development of peptic ulcer disease. (If emotional stress caused ulcers, we would *all* have them!) Stress ulcers are commonly seen in patients who are hospitalized for acute medical or surgical illnesses and are especially common in patients in the intensive care unit (ICU) being treated with mechanical ventilation. Stress ulcers probably arise from mucosal ischemia and loss of protective mechanisms, but the exact etiology of stress ulcers is often unclear. To further complicate matters, many patients in the ICU on mechanical ventilators require anticoagulating agents as part of the treatment of their underlying disease, which only compounds the problem of stress ulcers when they arise (ie, the heart attack that put you in the ICU on a ventilator is being treated in part via the use of blood thinners). When you develop a stress ulcer, the blood thinners reduce your ability to form a clot over the ulcer, and any bleeding that ensues can be brisker and more difficult to control.

- **Hypersecretory states:** In rare cases, tumors can stimulate acid production. These tumors, known as *gastrinomas*, can arise sporadically or in the context of certain genetic syndromes that give rise to many tumors. Gastrinomas, which produce the hormone gastrin in abundance and thus stimulate gastric acid production, can arise as part of multiple endocrine neoplasia type 1.

Types of Ulcers

There are many types of peptic ulcers that can develop. Peptic ulcers can arise in the stomach or the duodenum (usually in the first portion of the duodenum beyond the pylorus, known as the *duodenal bulb*). These can range from almost trivial breakdowns in the gastric or duodenal lining to ulcers with brisk, life-threatening arterial bleeding. An understanding of the different types of ulcers that can arise is helpful to clinicians because the ability to accurately recognize and describe a relevant lesion helps to guide treatment and suggests overall prognosis. The following is a list of the different types of lesions seen in peptic ulcer disease from the lowest to highest risk:

- **Erosions:** Erosions are the precursor lesions of ulcers. Erosions represent a small mucosal break, often with some surrounding inflammation.

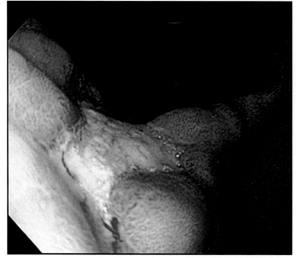

Figure 2-1. A large clean-based gastric ulcer seen on retroflexion.

Most erosions in the stomach and small bowel are asymptomatic, although they can produce microscopic blood loss. Most erosions are treated medically (eg, stopping NSAIDs, using acid-suppressing medications) and not endoscopically.

- **Clean-based ulcers:** Clean-based ulcers are among the most commonly encountered lesions in peptic ulcer disease. These are true ulcers that have a white and shiny base without signs of active or recent bleeding. Clean-based ulcers are also usually treated medically and rarely require endoscopic treatment (Figure 2-1).

- **Ulcers with flat pigmented spots:** Ulcers with flat pigmented spots are more suggestive of sites of recent bleeding. There is some disagreement on how best to manage patients with these lesions, with some endoscopists treating them aggressively during endoscopy and others opting for a more conservative approach focused on acid suppression.

- **Ulcers with an overlying clot:** Ulcers with an overlying clot are strongly suggestive of sources of bleeding. Often, it is possible to endoscopically remove the clot and treat any potential bleeding sources identified below.

- **Ulcers with a nonbleeding visible vessel:** Ulcers with a nonbleeding visible vessel are serious lesions that are very likely to bleed unless treated endoscopically. The name implies that an actual blood vessel can be seen in the ulcer bed.

- **Actively bleeding ulcers:** Actively bleeding ulcers are the most serious yet least frequently encountered lesions in peptic ulcer disease. Actively bleeding ulcers always warrant endoscopic therapy. These lesions have an open blood vessel that is actively leaking/spurting/spraying blood into the lumen.

- **Dieulafoy lesion:** A Dieulafoy lesion is not an ulcer per se, but it makes sense to discuss it here. A Dieulafoy lesion is a dilated submucosal vessel that can bleed spontaneously in the absence of an ulcer. The bleeding from these lesions can be massive and life-threatening. These are treated like ulcers with clips, sprays, and cautery.

Types of Endoscopic Therapy

Because peptic ulcer disease and gastrointestinal bleeding due to peptic ulcer disease are so incredibly common, a variety of endoscopic techniques to treat ulcers and stop bleeding have been developed. These techniques are often used in combination (ie, more than one endoscopic technique may be used in a single patient to treat a bleeding ulcer). New devices to treat peptic ulcer bleeding are constantly being developed, and over time, our armamentarium of weapons to stop these bleeds will likely only continue to expand. The following is a list of endoscopic therapies for ulcers:

- **Injection therapy:** Injection therapy refers to the use of a thin catheter with a needle at its tip, which is passed through an endoscope to inject certain agents into or around the base of the ulcer in an attempt to stop bleeding. In the United States, the most commonly used agent is diluted epinephrine. The primary role of injected agents is to produce mechanical tamponade of any nearby vessels via the creation of a submucosal fluid collection that extrinsically compresses the bleeding vessel. Injection therapy typically produces short-lived results and is rarely used in isolation for bleeding peptic ulcers. Injection therapy typically stops bleeding acutely so that the underlying ulcer can be washed and visualized more clearly in preparation for more definitive therapy (Figure 2-2).

- **Thermal therapy:** Thermal therapy refers to the use of devices passed through an endoscope that cause local heating of tissue in an attempt to cauterize bleeding or nonbleeding vessels in the ulcer. There are a variety of devices on the market that allow heat to be transmitted to tissue through an endoscope. Most of these rely on the use of electrocautery. It is worth noting that thermal therapy often relies on a process known as *coaptation*. Coaptation refers to the compression of the vessel in question by the probe before and during the application of thermal energy in an attempt to seal the vessel in a compressed/closed position and to minimize or stop bleeding altogether.

- **Mechanical therapy:** Mechanical therapy refers to the use of deployable objects to physically compress or close the vessel in an ulcer.

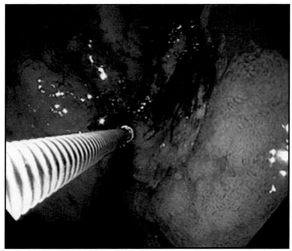

Figure 2-2. Injection of epinephrine solution into a gastric ulcer using a needle catheter.

Endoscopic clips represent the most commonly used form of mechanical therapy. Endoscopic clips, as their name implies, are small metal clips that can be deployed through an endoscope over ulcers and/or bleeding vessels in an attempt to stop bleeding. These clips are left behind, holding the blood vessel closed, when the endoscope is removed from the patient and can produce lasting hemostasis. Other forms of mechanical therapy include endoscopic loops or bands that can be placed around a bleeding ulcer as a sort of ligature. Clips and loops can be ideal for patients who use anticoagulation or antiplatelet medications because their function is not affected by blood-thinning agents (Figure 2-3). Some clips are narrow and thin and pass through the endoscope

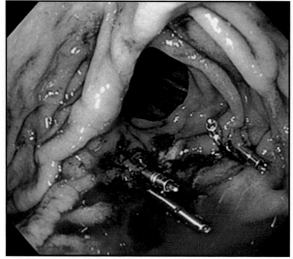

Figure 2-3. Four endoscopic clips applied to 2 ulcers in the stomach, with 2 clips applied to each ulcer.

(known as *through-the-scope clips*), and some are very large clips that fit over the end of the scope (known as *over-the-scope clips* [OTSCs]). OTSCs can close very large vessels or cover large areas of ulceration. OTSCs are so large they can also be used to close fistulas and some perforations!

- **Hemostatic powders:** Hemostatic powders can be sprayed to treat areas of bleeding. The powders themselves promote rapid clotting of blood. The powders come in canisters attached to endoscopic catheters that can be passed down an endoscope. Hemostatic powders are often used if the area of bleeding is large or diffuse or if the rate of bleeding is so great that the endoscopist cannot see well enough to do anything else. Hemostatic powders are usually not used alone. Rather, an endoscopist will use a hemostatic powder to slow or stop bleeding so that a second, more definitive technique (ie, clips) can be used additionally to provide a more durable hemostatic effect.

When treating patients with bleeding gastric ulcers, it has to be stressed that the endoscopic approach to these patients is just part of their overall care. Before endoscopy is undertaken, patients need to be stabilized from a hemodynamic point of view with fluid and blood resuscitation as needed through good intravenous (IV) access (generally described as *2 large bore IV lines* or a *central line*). Patients with poor blood clotting ability (coagulopathy) may need to have this corrected to help the bleeding to stop. IV proton pump inhibitors are started, and some patients may require ICU monitoring (and even mechanical ventilation) during a period of stabilization. Many/most patients are checked for *H pylori* infection and are treated if positive. Thus, endoscopy is a *piece* of the overall treatment plan and not the *entire* treatment plan in and of itself.

GASTRIC TUMORS

The stomach, like all organs in the gastrointestinal tract, is prone to develop neoplastic lesions, some of which are cancers. Tumors of the stomach can be separated into 2 groups: those of mucosal origin and those of submucosal origin. This refers to the fact that some tumors of the stomach arise from the innermost lining itself, whereas other lesions can arise from within the wall of the stomach from some of the deeper layers. Submucosal tumors can occur anywhere in the gastrointestinal tract but are very commonly encountered in the stomach. Thus, we can review submucosal lesions in this chapter.

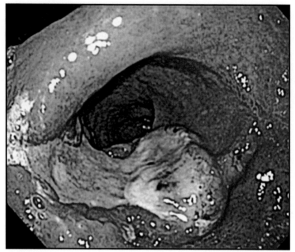

Figure 2-4. Large, ulcerated gastric cancer.

Tumors of Mucosal Origin

- Gastric adenocarcinoma is the most dreaded of all tumors of the stomach. Gastric adenocarcinoma is the fourth most common cancer worldwide and has a very high mortality rate. The most common risk factor for gastric adenocarcinoma is *H pylori* infection. *H pylori* probably lead to gastric adenocarcinoma through chronic inflammation over a long period of time. This chronic inflammation can lead to a state known as *metaplasia* in the gastric mucosa; metaplastic tissue is at high risk for undergoing malignant transformation to cancer (Figure 2-4). Gastric cancer may be associated with a more virulent form of *H pylori* infection that produces a protein known as *CagA* (cytotoxin-associated gene A). Other risk factors for gastric cancer include smoking, obesity, certain genetic syndromes (familial adenomatous polyposis and hereditary nonpolyposis syndrome), and diets high in N-nitroso compounds, which are commonly used as preservatives in foods, most notably smoked meats. Gastric cancer is relatively uncommon in Europe and North America, although it is extremely common throughout Asia, where gastric cancer screening programs are widespread. Sometimes the term *linitis plastica* is used to describe diffuse, infiltrating gastric cancer that results in a narrow, noncompliant stomach. Many patients with gastric adenocarcinoma present with advanced disease, and there are no surgical options for these patients. Early gastric cancers can be removed by endoscopic mucosal resection or endoscopic submucosal dissection using techniques similar to those described in Chapter 1. Gastric cancer is relatively rare in the West but very common in Asia. Most gastric cancers in Western countries are detected when they are advanced. In Asia, screening for gastric cancer is widespread, and many more early-stage tumors are discovered.

- Gastric carcinoids are neuroendocrine tumors that can arise from the gastric lining. Carcinoid tumors can also occur anywhere in the gastrointestinal tract but are very frequently encountered in the stomach as well as the small bowel. Carcinoid tumors originate from so-called *enterochromaffin-like cells*. Although these lesions actually do arise from the mucosa, they can mimic a submucosal lesion on endoscopy. Carcinoid tumors arise in a variety of settings, including Zollinger-Ellison syndrome, wherein a gastrin-secreting tumor of the stomach leads to excessive acid production, ulceration, and chronic atrophic gastritis. Small carcinoid tumors can be removed endoscopically;

if patients have multiple carcinoid tumors or the lesions are large, surgery is often recommended. Gastric carcinoids can develop in the setting of atrophic gastritis (a thinning of the lining of the stomach that can occur with age or in response to certain medications), certain tumor syndromes, or sporadically. Large gastric carcinoids can be removed surgically, but many small gastric carcinoids can be removed endoscopically via endoscopic mucosal resection or endoscopic submucosal dissection (Figure 2-5).

- Mucosa-associated lymphoid tissue (MALT) lymphoma (also known as *MALT-oma*) is a commonly encountered gastric malignancy. MALT lymphoma arises from B cells in the mucosa of the stomach. MALT lymphoma, even more so than gastric adenocarcinoma, is associated with *H pylori* infection. MALT lymphoma can mimic gastric adenocarcinoma when seen endoscopically, but simple cold forceps biopsy usually allows for determination between the 2 diseases. MALT lymphoma, like gastric adenocarcinoma, may be associated with more virulent forms of *H pylori* infection that produce CagA. Interestingly, early or low-grade MALT lymphomas can be treated with antibiotics alone in an effort to eradicate the underlying *H pylori* infection. This often results in complete eradication of the tumor. Patients with more advanced MALT lymphomas or early MALT lymphomas that fail to respond to *H pylori* eradication alone require additional therapies, most commonly chemotherapy.

Tumors of Submucosal Origin

- Lipomas are benign fatty tumors that are commonly encountered throughout the gastrointestinal

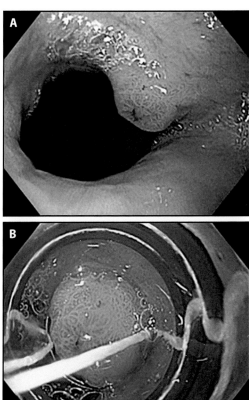

Figure 2-5. (A) A gastric carcinoid tumor referred for removal by endoscopic mucosal resection. (B) The carcinoid tumor is maneuvered into a cap on the tip of an endoscope. (*continued*)

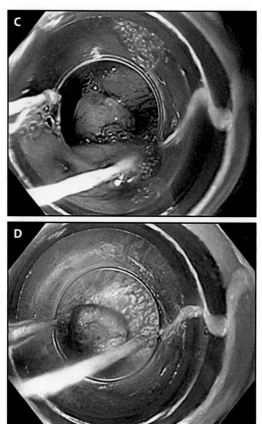

Figure 2-5 (continued). (C) An elastic band is deployed around the tumor, lifting it up from the surrounding stomach. (D) The tumor is removed using a snare with electrocautery. The resected tumor is now seen to have been severed from the gastric wall. Pathology showed complete removal.

tract and are often seen in the stomach. Lipomas can range from a few millimeters to several centimeters in size. Gastric lipomas often present as asymptomatic submucosal lesions detected during upper endoscopy. Typically, lipomas are very soft and deformable and have a yellowish color when viewed during upper endoscopy due to the color of the underlying fat. Most lipomas are true submucosal lesions that do not invade or distort the underlying muscularis propria of the bowel wall. On endoscopic ultrasound (EUS) examination, lipomas appear as bright hyperechoic lesions (Figure 2-6). This is a somewhat unique appearance; nothing else really looks like a lipoma. Rarely, lipomas can become symptomatic through one of two means. First, if a lipoma becomes large enough, it can cause obstruction of the stomach or bowel (depending on where it arises). If obstruction occurs, the lesion can usually be removed surgically without difficulty. Second, lipomas occasionally erode through the overlying mucosa of the bowel wall and bleed. Usually, it is easy to detect the fact that the lipoma is the source of the bleeding. If the bleeding cannot be controlled easily via endoscopic means, surgery is indicated. Malignant lesions known as *liposarcomas* have been seen in the stomach, although very rarely.

- Gastrointestinal stromal tumors (GISTs) are also very commonly encountered submucosal lesions of the gastrointestinal tract, and these are very frequently seen in the stomach. GISTs are unusual lesions in that they can be thought of as existing somewhere between benign and malignant with regard to their overall status. Small GISTs have a very low malignant potential, but these lesions can still give rise to metastases that behave in a malignant manner. Larger GISTs have a clearer

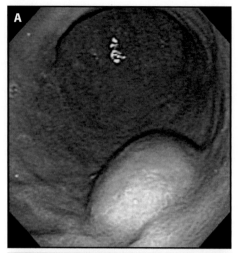

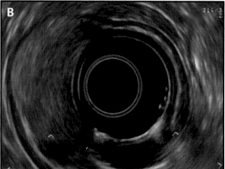

Figure 2-6. (A) Endoscopic view of a large submucosal lesion in the stomach. (B) 7.5-MHz EUS image of the same lesion as in A. Note the hyperechoic (bright) appearance to the lesion (arrow) consistent with a lipoma.

malignant potential and are often treated more aggressively. GISTs are mesenchymal in origin and often, but not always, stain positive for CD117, a tyrosine kinase receptor protein, and DOG1 (a special marker for GISTs). Many GISTs are asymptomatic, whereas others can present with a feeling of fullness in the abdomen, bleeding, or obstruction. On EUS, GISTs typically present as a hypoechoic, well-demarcated lesion that is seen to communicate with the muscularis propria, suggesting this as the wall layer of origin (Figure 2-7). GISTs are more likely to be malignant when they are large (greater than 3 cm), are heterogeneous in appearance on EUS, have internal cystic spaces, have irregular borders, and have many cells undergoing mitosis when viewed under a microscope. Interestingly, GISTs rarely spread to lymph nodes. The management of GISTs is somewhat tricky. Many patients are found to have small GISTs. These patients are often asymptomatic and elderly. It is often somewhat difficult for patients to accept surgery for a small lesion that is causing them no symptoms and may never cause them any harm. Larger lesions are often referred directly for surgery, whereas smaller lesions can either be removed or followed by endoscopy with or without EUS according to the patient's preference. Many patients with larger GISTs require long-term chemotherapy with tyrosine kinase inhibitor drugs, even after successful surgery. Sometimes GISTs are detected after they develop metastases. In these patients, chemotherapy and surgery are options, but these are rarely curative.

- Leiomyomas are benign tumors of smooth muscle origin that can be found in the stomach or, more commonly, the esophagus. Leiomyomas can mimic GISTs in appearance on EUS, and fine-needle

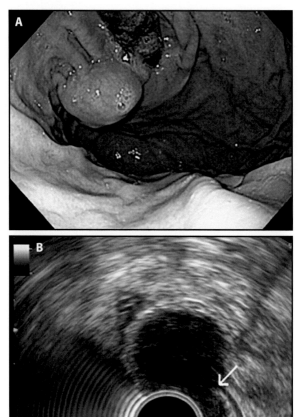

Figure 2-7. (A) Submucosal lesion in the gastric cardia seen on retroflexion. (B) 7.5-MHz EUS image of the lesion reveals a hypoechoic (dark) solid mass communicating with the muscularis propria (arrow) consistent with a GIST.

aspiration is often warranted to distinguish the 2 if there is uncertainty about the underlying diagnosis. Leiomyomas have very low malignant potential. Rarely, patients will be seen who have leiomyosarcomas, the malignant form of the disease. Most leiomyomas are asymptomatic, although large lesions can cause dysphagia (if they arise in the esophagus), abdominal fullness, or other symptoms. Leiomyomas may also appear to originate in or communicate with the muscularis propria, although leiomyomas (unlike GISTs) are generally negative on staining for CD117. Leiomyomas often stain positive for another marker known as *actin*. Asymptomatic leiomyomas do not require surgery as a general rule.

- A pancreatic rest usually appears as a submucosal lesion in the gastric antrum, often along the greater curvature in the prepyloric space. A pancreatic rest represents so-called *heterotopic pancreatic tissue*. What this really means is that the gastric wall contains some small amount of pancreatic tissue, completely separate from the nearby pancreas. These lesions are often umbilicated, which means they have a central opening or depression. Pancreatic rests are almost always asymptomatic in nature and can usually be definitively diagnosed just based on their appearance during upper endoscopy. If there is uncertainty about the diagnosis, EUS (with or without fine-needle aspiration) can be performed to investigate the lesion more closely. In general, a pancreatic rest requires no treatment.

- Duplication cysts can also be found throughout the gastrointestinal tract but are commonly encountered in the esophagus, stomach, and small bowel. Duplication cysts, as the name implies, form during embryogenesis and represent benign duplicated areas of the gastrointestinal tract. Interestingly, patients can also occasionally develop bronchogenic duplication cysts of pulmonary origin. Duplication cysts contain esophageal, gastric, or bowel wall as their lining and are often fluid and mucus filled. Duplication cysts have no malignant potential. In children, duplication cysts can cause abdominal pain or bowel obstruction and are often removed. In adults, duplication cysts are often asymptomatic lesions that do not require surgical resection. Rarely, they can become infected and require surgical drainage and/or removal.

- Extrinsic compression from another organ can often mimic a submucosal lesion. When patients undergo endoscopy, they are generally in the fasting state. If patients have an intact gallbladder, the fasting state will lead to a gallbladder that is full of bile. A full and distended gallbladder can often extrinsically compress the stomach and mimic a submucosal lesion. EUS can often readily identify that the area of concern is actually simply a healthy gallbladder. Similarly, the left lobe of the liver can sometimes compress the stomach and mimic a tumor. Rarely, gastric varices can mimic submucosal tumors as well.

GASTRIC ANTRAL VASCULAR ECTASIA

Gastric antral vascular ectasia (GAVE) is a relatively uncommon condition, but you need to know what it is and what to do about it when you come across it clinically. GAVE refers to the presence of neovascularization (the development of new blood vessels) in the stomach, almost always in the gastric antrum. These blood vessels are small, superficial, and often very numerous.

They often group in radial streaks and spread outward from the pylorus proximally through the antrum, and they can also manifest as small areas of punctate irregular blood vessels in the stomach that do not arise in streaks. GAVE is also referred to as *watermelon stomach* because some creative individual once thought that the linear streaks of GAVE appeared similar to a watermelon when viewed end on (I am not making this up!).

GAVE is most classically associated with liver disease, but it can be seen in several other diseases, including collagen vascular disorders, scleroderma, and chronic renal failure. Additionally, it can occur de novo in patients without any of these diseases.

GAVE can either be clinically silent or, more typically, can result in melena and/or occult gastrointestinal blood loss with resulting iron deficiency anemia. GAVE is treated via ablative methods to literally destroy the blood vessels and allow the mucosa to heal over. Argon plasma coagulation is the most common treatment for GAVE, but cryotherapy and radiofrequency ablation can be used as well. It often takes several sessions of endoscopic therapy to eradicate GAVE (Figure 2-8).

A Few Brief Words on Gastric Motility

Contractions of the musculature of the stomach are collectively referred to as *gastric motility*. You could write an entire textbook on gastric motility and the diseases that arise when this does not work properly (and, indeed, some people have!). However, for the purposes of this book, you should know that the stomach musculature receives innervation (a nerve supply) from a variety of sources, including the central nervous system, the vagus nerve, and the splanchnic nerves. The contractions of the

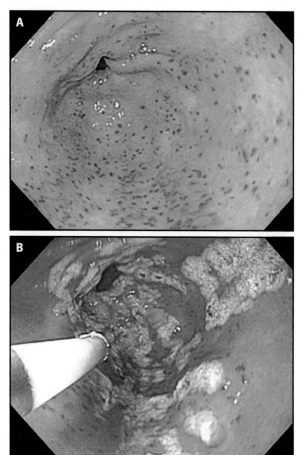

Figure 2-8. (A) GAVE. (B) Same patient as in A seen after argon plasma coagulation treatment to ablate GAVE.

stomach serve multiple functions. First, gastric contractions serve to mix food into homogeneous slurry that can be more easily digested. Second, gastric contractions serve to propel food through the pylorus and into the small bowel where digestion can continue.

In most people, gastric motility functions normally, and they happily go through their day digesting their meals without a second thought. However, there are many disorders of gastric motility, the most common of which is known as *gastroparesis*. The term *gastroparesis* specifically refers to a disorder of gastric motility wherein the stomach contracts and empties slowly, if at all. Patients with gastroparesis, most commonly diabetics in whom the nerves that regulate gastric motility have been damaged by prolonged exposure to high serum blood glucose concentrations, have a poorly contractile stomach that leads to symptoms such as nausea, vomiting, bloating, and abdominal pain. Gastroparesis in diabetic patients can further exacerbate poor glycemic control, which can worsen diabetes and, in turn, lead to worsening of the gastroparesis itself (a vicious cycle). Gastroparesis can also occur in a variety of other disease states and is often seen in patients who are taking chronic narcotic pain medications. These medications reduce gastrointestinal motility as a common side effect.

A variety of medications known as *promotility agents* are available to treat patients with gastroparesis. Some of these agents are antibiotics (ie, erythromycin) that have the side effect of promoting gastric motility, whereas others (ie, metoclopramide) are antiemetics that promote gastric motility directly.

Unfortunately, gastroparesis is a difficult disease to treat. Patients with gastroparesis are often typically advised to consume multiple small meals per day with a predominance of liquid or soft foods in an attempt to not overwhelm the stomach's limited capacity for gastric motility. Many patients have ongoing symptoms despite the use of medications and dietary modifications. Gastric pacemakers are available to electrically stimulate the stomach to contract, although these are not widely used at this time despite their appeal because there are limited data to show that they are effective in treating disorders of gastric motility. Another option is to inject botulinum toxin (Botox) into the pylorus (the muscular sphincter at the end of the stomach) to force it to relax and stay open for months at a time. The open pylorus lets food pass through much more easily. In my experience, Botox for gastroparesis is hit or miss in terms of giving patients relief, but it is worth trying because it is safe and easy to perform. Sometimes, if patients respond well to Botox, they can be referred to a surgeon to have their pylorus cut so it is permanently open, a procedure known as *pyloromyotomy*.

Two new treatments for gastroparesis exist that were not around a few years ago. The first of these is a so-called *gastric peroral endoscopic myotomy*. This is the same idea as the peroral endoscopic myotomy procedure discussed as a treatment for achalasia in Chapter 1 but is performed on the pylorus to cut the muscle permanently so that the pylorus stays open, thus allowing food to empty into the small bowel faster and easier (sort of like the way Botox works on the pylorus). Gastric peroral endoscopic myotomy is not practiced widely, but the limited data so far on its use are encouraging and the procedure can be considered in patients with severe gastroparesis.

Another new option for patients with gastroparesis, especially if they have a narrowed pylorus (known as *pyloric stenosis*), is to try to stent the pylorus open. This is usually done with a special stent known as a lumen-apposing metal stent (LAMS). LAMSs are very short stents that are fully covered and can be put across the pylorus to force it open to help the stomach empty faster and more efficiently (Figure 2-9). The advantages of an LAMS across the pylorus is that it can be quickly placed;

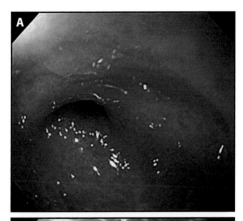

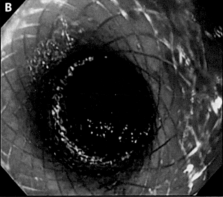

Figure 2-9. Use of an LAMS to treat gastroparesis in the setting of pyloric stenosis. The patient had severe gastroparesis from surgical transection of her vagus nerve. (A) Endoscopic image of the pylorus, showing a fixed, narrow opening. (B) Same patient after placement of an LAMS across the pylorus, showing that the opening is much wider and fixed in the open position. The patient had marked improvement of her symptoms.

is removable; and if the patient responds, it may suggest he or she should consider undergoing a more durable procedure to cut the pyloric musculature (ie, pyloromyotomy, as discussed earlier).

BIBLIOGRAPHY

Adler DG, Leighton JA, Davila RE, et al; American Society for Gastrointestinal Endoscopy. ASGE guideline: the role of endoscopy in acute non-variceal upper-GI hemorrhage. *Gastrointest Endosc.* 2004;60(4):497-504.

Gordon C, Kang JY, Neild PJ, Maxwell JD. The role of the hiatus hernia in gastro-oesophageal reflux disease. *Aliment Pharmacol Ther.* 2004;20(7):719-732.

Joensuu H, DeMatteo RP. The management of gastrointestinal stromal tumors: a model for targeted and multidisciplinary therapy of malignancy. *Annu Rev Med.* 2012;63:247-258.

Kahrilas PJ, Kim HC, Pandolfino JE. Approaches to the diagnosis and grading of hiatal hernia. *Best Pract Res Clin Gastroenterol.* 2008;22(4):601-616.

Ladeiras-Lopes R, Pereira AK, Nogueira A, et al. Smoking and gastric cancer: systematic review and meta-analysis of cohort studies. *Cancer Causes Control.* 2008;19(7):689-701.

Larson B, Adler DG. Lumen-apposing metal stents for gastrointestinal luminal strictures: current use and future directions. *Ann Gastroenterol.* 2019;32(2):141-146.

Pisters PW, Patel SR. Gastrointestinal stromal tumors: current management. *J Surg Oncol.* 2010;102(5):530-538.

Stathis A, Bertoni F, Zucca E. Treatment of gastric marginal zone lymphoma of MALT type. *Expert Opin Pharmacother.* 2010;11(13):2141-2152.

Chapter 3

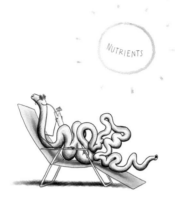

Small Intestine

ANATOMY AND PHYSIOLOGY

The main function of the small intestine is to absorb nutrients into systemic circulation. A normal adult can have approximately 18 to 20 feet of small intestine, with some individuals having more. To the naked eye, the small bowel looks like a long, tortuous, and floppy length of intestine that occupies much of the abdominal cavity.

In reality, the small bowel is divided both anatomically and physiologically into multiple segments that perform different functions. The small bowel is grossly covered internally by circular folds and is microscopically covered by finger-like projections that increase the

Adler DG. *The Little GI Book: An Easily Digestible Guide to Understanding Gastroenterology, Second Edition* (pp 71-98). © 2020 Taylor & Francis Group.

bowel's surface area tremendously and facilitate absorption of a variety of substances. From a structural point of view:

- The duodenum, which is the first segment of the small bowel, originates immediately after the pylorus and is broken up into 4 segments. The segments are referred to as the *first* (also known as the *bulb*), *second, third,* and *fourth portions of the duodenum.* The duodenal bulb is a somewhat chamber-like space that is used as an initial holding area for food transiting the pylorus from the stomach. The duodenal bulb ends at the "apex" and continues on to the second portion of the duodenum. The major and minor duodenal papillae are found in the second duodenum (Figure 3-1). The third and fourth portions of the duodenum, along with the second portion of the duodenum, are considered to be retroperitoneal structures; this means that they are not truly within the abdominal cavity. The small bowel terminates at the end of the fourth portion of the duodenum at the level of the ligament of Treitz. It is worth noting that the second, third, and fourth portions of the duodenum are all intimately associated with the pancreas.

- The second region of the small bowel is known as the *jejunum* (Figure 3-2). The jejunum is surrounded by mesentery, which is a double layer of the peritoneum that allows the small bowel to be mobile in the abdomen (ie, unlike organs like the pancreas and liver that occupy a fixed position, the small bowel has significant freedom of movement within the abdomen).

- The third portion of the small bowel is known as the *ileum.* The ileum is also surrounded by mesentery. The ileum connects the jejunum to the large intestine and terminates at the level of the

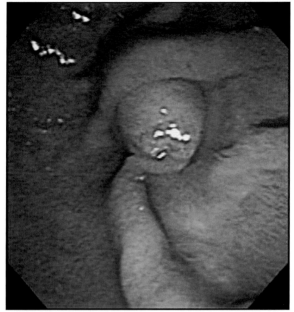

Figure 3-1. Normal major papilla in the second portion of the duodenum.

ileocecal valve. Of note, the most distal portion of the small bowel, just above the ileocecal valve, is referred to as the *terminal ileum*.

From a functional point of view:

- The duodenum helps to regulate the flow of gastric contents into the small bowel. Cells lining the duodenum release the hormone secretin, which stimulates the pancreas to secrete digestive enzymes and bicarbonate, and cholecystokinin, which stimulates the gallbladder to contract and release bile. Most of these pancreatic and biliary

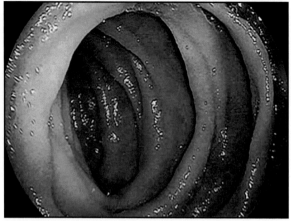

Figure 3-2. Normal-appearing small bowel in the jejunum.

secretions enter the duodenum via the major duodenal papilla, whose internal muscular structure, the sphincter of Oddi, relaxes in the face of these hormones to promote flow. Of note, iron is specifically absorbed in the duodenum.

- The jejunum is where much of the partially digested food from the stomach (now called *chyme*), enzymes, bicarbonate, and bile intermix, and food is further broken down into smaller molecules. Lipids (converted to fatty acids and glycerol), proteins (converted to amino acids), and carbohydrates (converted to oligosaccharides and monosaccharides) are actually absorbed through the small bowel wall and into the bloodstream. Some water is absorbed in the jejunum as well.

- The ileum is where absorption of the aforementioned breakdown products of food continues. In the terminal ileum specifically, bile salts manufactured in the liver and vitamin B_{12} are specifically reabsorbed. Patients who lose their ileum (either structurally due to trauma or surgery or functionally due to diseases that affect the ileum, such as Crohn's disease) can develop vitamin B_{12} deficiency and a specific type of diarrhea known as bile acid diarrhea (ie, if the patient cannot absorb the bile salts back into his or her circulation from the ileum and into the liver [via the so-called *enterohepatic circulation*], they pass into the colon where they can produce significant diarrhea). Bile acid diarrhea is usually treated by giving patients oral bile acid-binding agents (ie, cholestyramine), which often produce rapid improvement in diarrhea.

KEY DISEASES OF THE SMALL INTESTINE

Celiac Sprue (or Celiac Disease)

Celiac sprue refers to an immune intolerance for gluten proteins commonly found in wheat and related grains. Patients with celiac sprue specifically have an immune intolerance to gliadin, a component of gluten. These patients can have a range of symptoms from profound intractable diarrhea leading to severe malabsorption and death to an essentially asymptomatic state. Microscopically, the small bowel of patients with celiac sprue is noted to have a partial or total loss of villi (known as *villous atrophy*), as well as an extensive lymphocytic infiltrate consistent with a vigorous immune response to gluten-containing foods. Macroscopically, patients with celiac disease may have a notched appearance to their small bowel folds known as *scalloping*.

The story of celiac disease is interesting and worthy of a quick review; the ancients clearly described patients with celiac disease 2 millennia ago. In patients with profound symptoms, celiac sprue was often a death sentence because the disease itself was poorly understood and no specific treatment was available. Patients with celiac sprue often died of malabsorption and malnutrition despite eating voraciously. In the late 1800s, it was first noted that some patients could have relief of symptoms through the use of modified diets. In the 20th century, Willem Karel Dicke, a Dutch pediatrician, noticed that patients with celiac sprue improved clinically during World War II when there were a variety of shortages, most notably of wheat-containing products. After the war, when bread and other wheat-containing products became available again, Dicke noticed that patients with celiac sprue clinically worsened. Later work allowed Dicke and others to identify gluten and its component gliadin as the causative agents in patients with celiac sprue.

Patients with celiac sprue often have malabsorptive diarrhea with steatorrhea (fatty or greasy stools) and have difficulty maintaining their weight and their muscle mass. Patients often develop fat-soluble vitamin deficiencies as well as deficiencies in vitamin B_{12} and iron. Patients can also develop small intestine bacterial overgrowth (SIBO) due to poor small bowel function, and this can lead to an overall exacerbation of diarrhea and malabsorption. Iron deficiency and vitamin B_{12} deficiency can both lead to anemia, and unexplained anemia is a common indication to evaluate a patient for the presence or absence of celiac sprue. Patients with celiac sprue often develop itching from a blistering/vesicular rash on their extensor surfaces known as *dermatitis herpetiformis* (because it can mimic the appearance of cutaneous herpes infections). Celiac sprue puts patients at increased risk of developing small bowel adenocarcinoma or small bowel lymphoma (either B-cell or T-cell lymphoma).

Patients are diagnosed with celiac sprue via a variety of methods. The gold standard for diagnosis remains the identification of classic findings seen when looking at small bowel biopsies (obtained via esophagogastro-duodenoscopy) through a microscope. The biopsies should be obtained from patients with suspected celiac sprue who are consuming a diet that contains gluten. Additional blood tests often help to cement the diagnosis; these include positive testing for antigliadin and antiendomysial antibodies as well as positive testing for antitissue transglutaminase antibodies. Although duodenal biopsy remains the gold standard for diagnosis, patients often undergo blood testing first followed by endoscopy with biopsy to confirm the diagnosis. There is ongoing debate about how many small bowel biopsies should be obtained and from what points in the small intestine they should be obtained from in order to definitively attain or exclude the diagnosis of celiac sprue. In practice, most physicians obtain several biopsies from the second portion of the duodenum.

The hallmark of treatment of patients with celiac sprue is to initiate and maintain a gluten-free diet for life. Many patients discover rapidly how difficult it is to truly eat a gluten-free diet; gluten is everywhere in the modern Western diet. It is an incredible challenge to truly exclude gluten completely. Most patients with celiac sprue benefit from a formal evaluation by a nutritionist to help guide them toward a gluten-free diet, and, over time, patients can become very sophisticated at identifying gluten-free foods in the marketplace. Most patients who achieve a gluten-free or near gluten-free diet will have a marked and sustained improvement in their overall level of symptoms, and many become asymptomatic. Patients can relapse if they begin consuming gluten-containing foods, either intentionally or unintentionally. Adolescents with celiac sprue are historically difficult to treat because they are often noncompliant with a gluten-free diet (ie, it is hard not to eat some fast food with your friends once in a while when you are a teenager, even if you have celiac sprue and know that you should not).

Crohn's Disease

Crohn's disease is extremely important for you to understand. Crohn's disease is one of the two main forms of inflammatory bowel disease; ulcerative colitis (UC) is the other main form of inflammatory bowel disease. UC will be discussed in Chapter 4. Although Crohn's disease is known to affect the entire gastrointestinal tract, we will discuss it here because it is often primarily a disease of the small intestine.

The key features of Crohn's disease to be aware of include the following:

- Crohn's disease is best described as an inflammatory disorder of the gastrointestinal tract that results in transmural inflammation (ie, the inflammation extends all the way through the bowel wall and thus involves all of the layers of the bowel wall).

- Endoscopically, patients with Crohn's disease often have linear or serpiginous ulcers (Figure 3-3) and/or what are referred to as *aphthous ulcers*. Aphthous ulcers appear as discrete round-to-oval ulcers in the gastrointestinal tract. Patients with Crohn's disease often also develop these aphthous ulcers in their mouths. These oral ulcers can range from painless to a source of excruciating pain.

- Severe inflammation in patients with Crohn's disease can lead to the formation of deep ulcers referred to as *fissures* or penetrating lesions known as *fistulas*. Fistulas are through-and-through erosions/ulcerations involving the entire bowel wall where a communication ("hole") forms between a loop of the small bowel and some other structure (another loop of the small bowel, bladder, colon, vagina, or even the skin, resulting in a so-called *enterocutaneous fistula*).

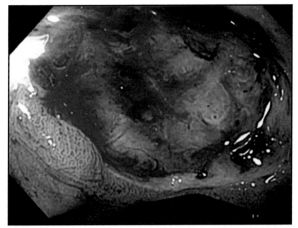

Figure 3-3. Deep small bowel ulcer in a patient with Crohn's disease.

- Although Crohn's disease can affect the entire gastrointestinal tract, the small bowel, especially the terminal ileum, is most commonly affected.
- Crohn's disease can involve the colon and can produce a form of colitis known as *Crohn's colitis.*
- Biopsies of the bowel from patients with Crohn's disease often reveal noncaseating granulomas.
- Crohn's disease is typically discontinuous (ie, areas of a diseased bowel are often interspersed with a normal-appearing and normal-functioning bowel).
- Crohn's disease is associated with growing up in conditions of better hygiene, possibly resulting from limited or delayed exposure to pathogens during childhood.
- Crohn's disease is often a disease of current smokers (in contrast to UC, which is often a disease of former smokers).

- Crohn's disease is more commonly encountered in Ashkenazi Jews.
- There is a strong genetic component to Crohn's disease with individuals from families that have members with inflammatory bowel disease more likely to develop Crohn's disease or UC themselves. Recent studies have identified a gene on chromosome 16 referred to as *NOD2* that has been associated with the development of Crohn's disease.
- Despite all of this, it should be stressed that there is no clear cause for Crohn's disease in all patients, and the disease is still considered idiopathic in nature.

Common clinical features of Crohn's disease include the following:

- Abdominal pain, most commonly in the right lower quadrant
- Frequent diarrhea that is usually nonbloody (unless there is colonic involvement)
- Abdominal cramping
- Fevers
- Perianal disease in the form of fissures, fistulas, and abscesses. Abscesses are often intra-abdominal or perianal. Perianal abscesses are a severe complication of Crohn's disease and often require combined medical and surgical treatment.
- Extraintestinal manifestations of Crohn's disease are common. These can also be seen in patients with UC. Extraintestinal manifestations of inflammatory bowel disease to look for include the following:
  - Oral ulcers
  - Skin ulcers known as *pyoderma gangrenosum* (which can be severe)
  - Erythema nodosum, a dermatologic disorder in which patients develop inflamed painful nodules along their extremities, often along the extensor surfaces

- Peripheral arthropathy or arthritis of either small or large joints
- Ankylosing spondylitis, a type of arthritis that affects portions of the lower spine and the sacroiliac joints
- Ocular complications including scleritis and episcleritis as well as uveitis
- Kidney stones from disordered oxalate metabolism in patients with distal small bowel (ileal) disease
- Gallstones from disordered bile salt metabolism in patients with distal small bowel (ileal) disease
- Primary sclerosing cholangitis (a chronic inflammatory disease of the bile ducts; this is discussed extensively in Chapter 6)
- Amyloidosis (this is rare but has been described, often in patients with Crohn's disease)
- Vitamin and mineral deficiencies from malabsorption and maldigestion

Patients with Crohn's disease run the gamut from a well and completely asymptomatic state to a severely debilitated state in which patients cannot live on their own outside of a hospital setting. As a general rule, the goals of treatment in patients with Crohn's disease include controlling underlying gastrointestinal inflammation, inducing clinical remission, preventing disease flare-ups, and treating any extraintestinal manifestations. It should be stressed that the treatment of Crohn's disease involves both medical and surgical management. Most patients can be managed through the proper administration of medications, although many patients will ultimately require some form of surgery (either to drain abscesses, correct fistulas, and/or remove areas of a severely diseased bowel). In patients with Crohn's disease, it is imperative for them to keep as much functioning small bowel as possible; repeated surgeries can lead to short bowel syndrome (in which the patient no longer has enough functioning small bowel to adequately absorb nutrients).

Medications for treating Crohn's disease can be given alone or in combination. Some key medications used to treat Crohn's disease (and UC) include the following:

- **Corticosteroids:** These agents can be given to patients orally or intravenously. Steroids are often very effective agents in treating patients with Crohn's disease and can produce a dramatic improvement in symptoms and induce clinical remission. Patients may have difficulties tapering off of these medications without having a flare of their disease. The side effects of steroids include weight gain, a puffy or moonlike face, acne, and emotional disturbances, such as depression or anxiety. In severe cases, steroid use can lead to suicidal thoughts. Fortunately, this is rare. Steroid use can also lead to suppression of the patient's adrenal gland (where endogenous corticosteroids are manufactured), and steroid medications should be tapered slowly in patients who have experienced long-standing steroid treatment to prevent adrenal insufficiency and to give the adrenal glands sufficient time to "wake up" and begin producing endogenous corticosteroids again. It is of note that corticosteroids are less effective at maintaining remission than inducing it in patients with Crohn's disease. Budesonide is an oral steroid that is metabolized rapidly as the drug passes through the liver for the first time after absorption and has fewer systemic side effects than most other corticosteroids. Budesonide is often very helpful in patients with ileal disease because the drug is very effective in treating inflammation in the distal small bowel. Budesonide is not typically used for treating Crohn's colitis.

- **Antibiotics:** Antibiotics have been used to treat Crohn's disease (and, to a lesser extent, UC) for many years. The most commonly used antibiotics for patients with Crohn's disease include ciprofloxacin and metronidazole. These antibiotics are generally used in patients with fistulas, abscesses, or perianal Crohn's disease. These drugs may also be of value in patients with Crohn's colitis. A new addition to the antibiotic market, rifaximin, has also been used in Crohn's disease. This drug has the advantage of being very poorly absorbed, so it stays active within the bowel lumen for a long period of time.

- **Nonsteroidal immunosuppressive drugs:** This class of medications is most notably includes azathioprine and 6-mercaptopurine (6-MP). Azathioprine and 6-MP are often better tolerated over the long term than corticosteroids and are frequently used to help induce and maintain remission in patients with Crohn's disease. The use of these agents requires careful patient monitoring to ensure that there is not excessive suppression of the patient's immune system (which could lead to infections). In addition, there is heterogeneity in how rapidly patients metabolize these 2 agents, which affects their dosing based on the different genes patients harbor for an enzyme known as *thiopurine methyltransferase*. Thiopurine methyltransferase gene testing is commonly performed in patients receiving azathioprine or 6-MP. Other nonsteroidal immunosuppressive drugs include cyclosporine and methotrexate. Cyclosporine is more commonly used in refractory UC than in Crohn's disease, whereas methotrexate (a folate inhibitor) is more commonly used in patients with Crohn's disease. The long-term use of methotrexate is associated with liver fibrosis, and patients using this drug need to be monitored for liver disease over time. Liver fibrosis in patients using methotrexate is dose dependent, and patients with higher cumulative doses of the drug are at increased risk for liver injury.

- **Biologics (also known as** *biologic agents*): The term *biologics*, when used within the context of inflammatory bowel disease, refers to a class of drugs that are not medications in the typical sense of the word; these agents are biologically active antibodies given to patients with inflammatory bowel disease in an attempt to modulate their immune system and thus reduce symptoms. Some of these agents function as antibodies to the human humoral factor known as *tumor necrosis factor* (TNF) and are often referred to as *anti-TNF antibodies*. There are 3 anti-TNF antibodies commercially available: infliximab, certolizumab, and adalimumab. Biologics are very powerful medications that can often bring about a rapid and sustained response in patients with otherwise difficult to treat inflammatory bowel disease. These drugs are primarily used to treat patients with Crohn's disease, although they can play a role in patients with UC as well. Biologic agents are especially helpful in patients with fistulizing Crohn's disease. Biologic agents are often used in combination with another immunosuppressive drug; this enhances the efficacy of the treatment overall and can help minimize the formation of antibodies to these agents themselves (ie, antibodies to infliximab). Biologics must be used carefully; patients using these agents are at risk for infection or for reactivation of hepatitis B or tuberculosis. As such, testing for pre-existing hepatitis B or tuberculosis is recommended before initiating treatment with biologic agents.

- The following are some details about biologics for Crohn's disease (the names take some getting used to):

  - Infliximab was the first biologic. It is a monoclonal antibody against TNF. Infliximab is made of both human and murine (mouse) elements combined into one antibody. Infliximab is administered via intravenous infusion.

  - Certolizumab is a monoclonal antibody fragment that acts against TNF. Certolizumab is bound to a molecule known as *polyethylene glycol* that helps to increase its half-life. Certolizumab is administered via subcutaneous injection.

  - Adalimumab is also a monoclonal antibody against TNF. Adalimumab is administered via subcutaneous injection.

- **Biosimilars:** Biosimilars are drugs that are very, very close to the molecular structure of biologics. Biosimilars are thought to have very similar, if not the same, activity when used in patients with Crohn's disease (and UC; see Chapter 4). A dozen biosimilars have been approved for use in the United States, with several of them being biosimilars for treating inflammatory bowel disease. In general, biosimilars are cheaper than biologics.

- **Aminosalicylates:** Aminosalicylates are a group of drugs widely used in the treatment of inflammatory bowel disease. The molecule 5-aminosalicylic acid (5-ASA), known as *mesalamine*, is the active agent in these medications. 5-ASA works as a topical anti-inflammatory in the bowel. Aminosalicylates are available in many formulations, including oral capsules (typically used for small bowel and proximal colon inflammation) and rectal suppositories, enemas, and foams (for distal colonic inflammation).

Small Intestine Bacterial Overgrowth

SIBO is a common cause of diarrhea that originates from the small bowel. In most patients, the small bowel is relatively free of bacteria when compared with the large intestine (which is loaded with bacteria). Patients with SIBO have an abnormal and pathologic increase in the concentration of small bowel bacteria. SIBO can arise in a variety of other clinical settings; these typically involve some baseline abnormality in small bowel structure and/ or function. The classic disorder that gives rise to SIBO is diabetes mellitus. Patients with diabetes develop a visceral enteropathy, which results in poor small bowel contractions (similar to what happens in the stomach in diabetics with gastroparesis). These poor small bowel contractions result in reduced clearing of bacteria from the small bowel and can lead to SIBO. Other conditions that can give rise to SIBO include celiac disease, scleroderma, the use of immunosuppressive drugs, and postsurgical anatomy. Postsurgical anatomy can give rise to SIBO through the loss of normal anatomic structure and function; SIBO can be seen in patients after bariatric surgery, loss of the ileocecal valve, and pancreaticobiliary surgery with associated small bowel reconstruction. For unclear reasons, SIBO can occasionally be seen in patients without any obvious risk factors.

Patients with SIBO most commonly present with chronic diarrhea and weight loss but can also develop abdominal pain, dyspepsia, nausea, vomiting, and bloating. Patients can also develop vitamin B_{12} deficiency (which can lead to a macroscopic anemia), iron-deficiency anemia (which can lead to microcytic anemia), and deficiency of the fat-soluble vitamins A, D, E, and K.

SIBO can be diagnosed via a variety of methods. Direct aspiration of fluid from the duodenum (obtained during upper endoscopy) can be cultured and quantified. If the bacterial load is calculated to be greater than 10^5 bacteria/cc, most would consider this to be diagnostic for SIBO. A variety of breath tests are available to test for SIBO. Most of the available breath tests involve ingestion of radiolabeled carbohydrates with measurements of exhaled breath at various time points after ingestion. The appearance of radiolabeled carbon dioxide in exhaled breath at certain time points after ingestion suggests that SIBO has occurred and bacteria in the small bowel are breaking down the radiolabeled carbohydrates.

The mainstay of treatment for SIBO is a course of antibiotics, generally 5 to 14 days in duration. There are no hard and fast guidelines on which antibiotics to use to treat SIBO; fluoroquinolones, metronidazole, or penicillin-based antibiotics are commonly used. Rifaximin and neomycin are also viable alternatives. Most patients with SIBO will have a rapid response to antibiotic therapy with improvement in their symptoms, most notably diarrhea. The interval at which patients with SIBO need to be retreated is highly variable. The antibiotics will succeed in eradicating the SIBO, but, as a rule, the underlying condition that led to the SIBO in the first place is likely still present, and the small bowel will be recolonized with bacteria over time, resulting in a return of SIBO symptoms. As a rule, I let patients tell me when they feel that they need another course of antibiotics. Some patients can go only a few weeks between courses of antibiotics, whereas other patients with less severe SIBO only require antibiotic treatment once or twice a year to maintain good control of their symptoms. As a general rule, you do not want to use the same drug over and over again in patients with SIBO; this could lead to resistant bacterial strains. It is a good idea to rotate between several drugs to prevent the development of resistance (ie, first, treat the patient with 1 week of an oral fluoroquinolone, then metronidazole, and then amoxicillin).

In practice, I rarely order small bowel bacterial counts or breath tests to diagnose patients with suspected SIBO. If the patient has a history and symptoms compatible with SIBO or if he or she has an obvious risk factor for SIBO (eg, scleroderma, diabetes), I will often simply treat the patient with an empiric trial of antibiotics. If the patient responds to antibiotics, you have essentially confirmed the diagnosis of SIBO and now have a treatment plan for going forward. If the patient does not respond to a trial of antibiotics, you might need to rethink the diagnosis and perform other investigations.

Small Bowel Cancer

Primary small bowel cancer, which is most commonly adenocarcinoma, is rarely encountered clinically. As with most gastrointestinal cancers, small bowel adenocarcinoma can be seen in the setting of chronic inflammation over a prolonged period of time. Diseases that can lead to chronic small bowel inflammation include celiac disease and Crohn's disease. Other diseases that can give rise to small bowel adenocarcinoma include the polyposis syndromes Peutz-Jeghers syndrome and familial adenomatous polyposis. Other tumors that can arise in the small bowel include carcinoid tumors and lymphomas. Most patients with small bowel cancer of any kind will present with bleeding and/or obstructive symptoms. In some cases, a small bowel perforation will be the first manifestation of disease. Weight loss, anemia, or nonspecific findings may precede more overt symptoms of malignancy. The mainstay of treatment for patients with small bowel adenocarcinoma or carcinoid tumors is surgery. Stents can be used to relieve bowel obstruction in patients who are not surgical candidates (Figure 3-4). Lymphomas are generally treated with chemotherapy.

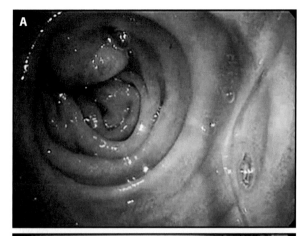

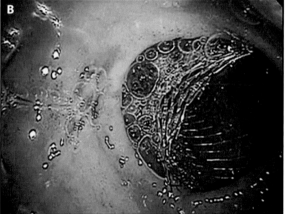

Figure 3-4. (A) Near-obstructing small bowel adenocarcinoma. (B) Same patient as in A, now with placement of a small bowel stent to relieve obstructive symptoms.

Diarrhea of Small Bowel Origin

Many patients develop diarrhea of small bowel origin, and this can be acute or chronic. Diarrhea of small bowel origin can arise through the following mechanisms:

- **Infections:** Many conditions that lead to diarrhea affect the small bowel. Diarrhea of small bowel origin can be infectious, traumatic, osmotic, secretory, or inflammatory in nature.

  Infectious diarrhea is usually caused by bacteria or viruses. Patients can acquire food or waterborne illness such as *Salmonella, Shigella, Escherichia coli, Vibrio cholera, Campylobacter jejuni, Giardia* (a parasite), and other pathogens, either through normal daily exposures or through unusual exposures during travel. Patients often present with acute diarrheal illness associated with an unusual food exposure (eg, eating at a county fair, travel to a foreign country), although they may have no unusual food exposures at all. Some of these infections (ie, cholera) result in diarrhea due to a toxin produced by the infectious organism. These toxins can affect the bowel's ability to absorb and/or secrete fluid and electrolytes into the bowel lumen, resulting in diarrhea. Other infections (*Salmonella* and *Shigella*) produce diarrhea by direct invasion of the small bowel with a resulting loss of functional small bowel surface and the inability to properly absorb fluid and nutrients.

  Immunocompromised patients (including patients with HIV/AIDS and patients taking immunosuppressive medications, such as organ or bone marrow transplant recipients) can develop infectious diarrhea from such parasites as *Isospora belli, Cryptosporidium*, and microsporidia; viruses such as herpes simplex virus; or other pathogens such as *Mycobacterium avium* complex. These infections are rarely seen in immunocompetent hosts.

- **Secretory diarrhea:** Secretory diarrhea occurs when some agent is specifically stimulating the bowel to produce or release fluid and electrolytes into the lumen, resulting in diarrhea. Secretory diarrhea can be infectious in nature (as is the case with the cholera toxin discussed previously) or may be related to other causes, such as tumors. Neuroendocrine tumors, including glucagonoma, carcinoid tumors, vasoactive intestinal peptide secreting tumors, and somatostatinomas, are all associated with diarrhea.

- **Short bowel syndrome:** Short bowel syndrome refers to patients who have malabsorptive diarrhea due to insufficient small bowel surface area from a variety of causes. Patients can develop short bowel syndrome from any illness that warrants extensive small bowel resection. Some examples would include patients who undergo small bowel resections for Crohn's disease, abdominal trauma, or small bowel obstructions and/or volvulus where significant amounts of bowel are no longer viable and are removed. Patients can also develop functional short bowel syndrome in the setting of severe Crohn's disease without a history of surgery where the bowel is simply so inflamed that it can no longer function. Bariatric surgeries often intentionally produce anatomic reconstructions that create a functional short bowel syndrome. The most common bariatric surgery, the Roux-en-Y gastric bypass, limits the size of the gastric lumen through gastric reconstruction and also dramatically reduces the amount of small bowel available for nutrient absorption (producing a catabolic state, resulting in weight loss). Some patients with Roux-en-Y gastric bypass can develop diarrhea similar to that seen in short bowel syndrome. Patients with short bowel syndrome may require specialized diets and/or eating habits (multiple small meals per day) in an attempt to better use what functional small bowel they have. Some patients with short bowel syndrome simply do not have enough small bowel to maintain their weight and absorb adequate nutrients. These patients are often treated with total parenteral nutrition intravenously or, more rarely, undergo small bowel transplantation. Experimental techniques exist whereby a patient's own small bowel can be functionally lengthened to increase the surface area, but these are performed only at specialized centers.

- **Motility disorders:** Patients with disordered small bowel motility can commonly develop diarrhea. Patients with diabetes mellitus often develop visceral neuropathy and can develop so-called *diabetic diarrhea* due to rapid transit of food to the small bowel with inadequate time for absorption of fluid, electrolytes, and nutrients. Patients with hyperthyroidism can have hypercontractility of the small bowel that can lead to diarrhea as well.

- **Osmotic diarrhea:** Osmotic diarrhea develops when patients ingest an agent that is either nonabsorbable or poorly absorbable that results in fluid being drawn into or retained in the small bowel lumen via osmotic forces. Osmotic diarrhea is typically caused by the ingestion of ions such as magnesium, sulfate, and phosphate (commonly used in laxatives) or sugars that are difficult for the body to break down such as mannitol, lactulose, and sorbitol (also used in laxatives). Patients who are lactose intolerant and who lack the enzyme lactase can develop osmotic diarrhea when eating lactose-containing foods, such as milk or ice cream. Patients may ingest these osmotic agents intentionally (ie, the patient who buys a bottle of magnesium citrate from a pharmacy to treat his or her constipation is attempting to induce osmotic diarrhea on purpose). Other patients with osmotic diarrhea may be ingesting these substances unwittingly (ie, many dietary candies use sorbitol as a sweetener). Patients eating these candies may not realize that their subsequent diarrhea is caused by the sorbitol that they are ingesting. Patients with anorexia nervosa often attempt to lose weight through laxative abuse, often via the use of laxatives that produce osmotic diarrhea. Patients with hepatic encephalopathy are commonly treated with lactulose to induce osmotic diarrhea (see Chapter 5 for more details).

- **Inflammatory diarrhea:** Inflammatory diarrhea can come from chronic inflammation of the small bowel lumen, most commonly from Crohn's disease. Patients undergoing chemotherapy and/or radiation therapy can also develop small bowel inflammation that results in diarrhea.

- **Functional disorders producing diarrhea:** Irritable bowel syndrome (IBS) is a chronic abdominal condition in which patients can experience abdominal pain, bloating, and disorders of bowel function, including constipation and/or diarrhea. IBS is considered a syndrome rather than a true disease; no universally agreed upon and clear cause has been identified for IBS. Patients can develop constipation-predominant IBS, diarrhea-predominant IBS (IBS-D), or IBS with alternating constipation and diarrhea. Some patients may have abdominal pain only. IBS-D is common. These patients have chronic diarrhea that defies investigations without evidence of infection, secretory diarrhea, osmotic diarrhea, etc. Patients with IBS-D can be treated with high-fiber diets (to increase the bulk of their stools) as well as agents such as loperamide or opiates to slow bowel contractility. It can be difficult to completely resolve diarrhea in patients with IBS-D. It is also worth noting that many patients without true IBS will experience diarrhea during times of extreme stress; this often goes away when the underlying stressful situation resolves.

- **Medication side effects:** Many medications can cause diarrhea as a side effect. These agents may affect the small bowel, the large bowel, or both. It seems most appropriate to discuss them here under small bowel diarrhea. Patients may often recognize that the medication is causing diarrhea, given a temporal relationship between the development of diarrhea and the initiation of the drug. Conversely, patients may not recognize any association or may be unable to tell you about such an association (eg, institutionalized patients, patients with dementia). It is always worth mentioning to patients and/or their caregivers the potential for diarrhea in medications you prescribe if the possibility exists.

Medications that have been associated with causing diarrhea include the following:

  - Proton pump inhibitors
  - H2 receptor antagonists
  - Antibiotics
  - Selective serotonin reuptake inhibitor antidepressants
  - Antacids
  - Antibiotics

- ◦ Cardiac medications (especially antiarrhythmic agents)
- ◦ Colchicine (used to treat gout)
- ◦ Theophylline
- ◦ Nonsteroidal anti-inflammatory drugs
- ◦ 5-ASA agents

Small Bowel Bleeding

Although most gastrointestinal bleeding comes from either the foregut (the esophagus, stomach, and duodenum) or the colon, a small subset of patients will have bleeding from the small intestine. These patients can have active, brisk bleeding but more often than not have low-level, chronic blood loss that leads to anemia. Of note, small bowel bleeding visible to the patient is called *overt bleeding*, whereas blood loss that the patient cannot see is referred to as *occult bleeding*. If common causes of gastrointestinal bleeding have been ruled out and the small bowel needs to be investigated, endoscopy is usually in order. If endoscopy fails to find the source of bleeding, other investigations including special x-ray scans, angiography, or even surgery can be required.

Different types of special endoscopic procedures are required to investigate the small bowel (see Chapter 8 for details). The reason special endoscopes are needed is because the small bowel is very long, tortuous (twisty), and difficult to access.

Common causes of small bowel bleeding include the following:

- • **Arteriovenous malformations (AVMs):** AVMs are superficial, fragile blood vessels that can form spontaneously or can arise due to other medical conditions or in the setting of the use of certain medications (Figure 3-5). AVMs are very

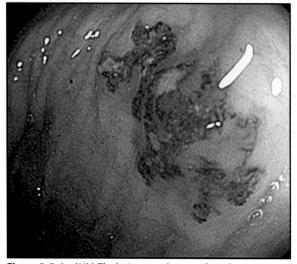

Figure 3-5. An AVM. The lesion was destroyed via electrocautery.

commonly found in patients with bleeding of small bowel origin. AVMs are generally destroyed by cautery when found.

- **Ulcers:** Just as in other parts of the gastrointestinal tract, ulcers (often from nonsteroidal anti-inflammatory drugs or unsuspected inflammatory bowel disease) can cause bleeding in the small bowel.
- **Polyps:** Polyps can form sporadically or as part of certain polyp syndromes (discussed previously).
- **Tumors:** Small bowel tumors are rare but can include adenocarcinoma, lymphoma, carcinoid tumors, and metastases.
- **Meckel's diverticulum:** This refers to a diverticulum (pocket) in the small bowel that contains acid-producing gastric mucosa. These lesions

cannot bleed; have low-level bleeding; or result in a massive, life-threatening gastrointestinal bleeding event. Meckel's diverticulum can be identified on endoscopy, on a special nuclear medicine test known as a *Meckel's scan*, during angiography, or during surgery. Most symptomatic Meckel's diverticula are surgically removed.

- **Dieulafoy lesion:** These are abnormal, submucosal vessels that can spontaneously bleed. They can also occur in the stomach. Most are treated via endoscopy or angiography.
- **Kaposi's sarcoma:** This is a tumor often seen in patients with untreated HIV/AIDS.
- **Hemobilia:** Bleeding from the bile duct that enters the small bowel via the ampulla can often be confused for primary small bowel bleeding.
- **Hemosuccus pancreaticus:** Bleeding from the pancreatic duct that enters the small bowel via the ampulla can also be confused for primary small bowel bleeding.
- There are many other causes of small bowel bleeding, usually involving rare tumor syndromes.

BIBLIOGRAPHY

Abraham B, Sellin JH. Drug-induced diarrhea. *Curr Gastroenterol Rep*. 2007;9(5):365-372.

Cottone M, Renna S, Orlando A, Mocciaro F. Medical management of Crohn's disease. *Expert Opin Pharmacother*. 2011;12(16):2505-2525.

Dicke WK, Weijers NA, Van De Kamer JH. Coeliac disease. II. The presence in wheat of a factor having a deleterious effect in cases of Coeliac disease. *Acta Paediatr*. 1953;42(1):34-42.

Eusufzai S. Bile acid malabsorption: mechanisms and treatment. *Dig Dis*. 1995;13(5):312-321.

Kupper C. Dietary guidelines and implementation for celiac disease. *Gastroenterology*. 2005;128(4 Suppl 1):S121-S127.

Lichtenstein GR, Hanauer SB, Sandborn WJ; Practice Parameters Committee of American College of Gastroenterology. Management of Crohn's disease in adults. *Am J Gastroenterol*. 2009;104(2):465-483; quiz 464, 484.

Schuppan D, Junker Y, Barisani D. Celiac disease: from pathogenesis to novel therapies. *Gastroenterology*. 2009;137(6):1912-1933.

Chapter 4

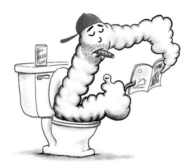

Colon and Rectum

As the least glamorous of all the gastrointestinal organs, the colon and rectum are nonetheless vitally important for digestive health. Colorectal diseases are extremely common in gastroenterology, and you will likely spend a disproportionate amount of your time caring for patients with diseases of these organs. With the widespread adoption of screening colonoscopy programs to reduce the risk of colorectal cancer, an awareness of the importance of the colon and rectum in normal health and disease has become central to modern gastroenterology.

Adler DG. *The Little GI Book: An Easily Digestible Guide to Understanding Gastroenterology, Second Edition* (pp 99-126). © 2020 Taylor & Francis Group.

FUNCTION

The primary function of the colon is to absorb water from its lumen. This removal of water allows for the formation of concentrated solid stools. This explains why many colonic diseases result in diarrhea; if the colon cannot adequately absorb water from stool, then diarrhea, with its accompanying loss of fluids and electrolytes, must ensue. Similarly, the colon plays a small role in the absorption of sodium and other substances, such as the fat-soluble vitamin K.

The rectum primarily serves as a reservoir for stool. This reservoir allows you to retain stool within your body until such time as it is appropriate to have a bowel movement. Rectal diseases often result in incontinence and/or what is referred to as *urgency*. Urgency refers to the need to have a bowel movement immediately.

ANATOMY

Colonic anatomy is relatively straightforward (Figure 4-1). The terminal ileum joins the most proximal portion of the colon, known as the *cecum*, at the ileocecal valve. The valve prevents backflow of colonic contents into the small bowel. The cecum, somewhat similar to the rectum, is a chamber whose role is to accommodate the contents of the small bowel as they first enter the colon. The cecum also contains the appendiceal orifice, which, as its name implies, opens to the lumen of the appendix itself. Passing distally from the cecum above the ileocecal valve is the ascending colon. This region of bowel is so named because it ascends from the right lower quadrant in the pelvis to the right upper quadrant of the abdomen. The ascending colon terminates at the level of the hepatic flexure. The hepatic flexure is a bend in the large bowel that occurs along the underside of

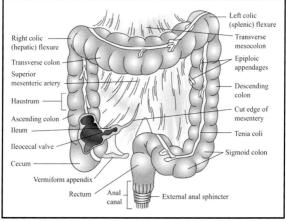

Figure 4-1. Diagram of the colon showing key anatomic aspects.

the liver. During colonoscopy, one can almost always see the blue shadow of the liver abutting the large bowel itself. Moving distally, the next region of the large bowel is known as the *transverse colon*. The transverse colon passes from the right upper quadrant to the left upper quadrant and is remarkable for its triangular-shaped lumen. The transverse colon ends at the level of the splenic flexure. As its name would imply, this is where the colon abuts the spleen and makes a sharp turn inferiorly to become the descending colon. The descending colon moves from the left upper quadrant down to the pelvis and terminates at the level of the sigmoid colon. The sigmoid colon, as its name would imply, is often a region of highly torturous large bowel in the left lower quadrant. The sigmoid colon terminates at the level of the rectum. The rectum itself is generally defined as the final 12 to 15 cm of the large bowel. Below the rectum is the anal sphincter complex and the anus itself.

It is worth making the comment that, although the previous description makes the anatomy of the large bowel look very simple and straightforward, in reality few patients have a colon that looks like the one in the accompanying drawing. A typical barium enema will illustrate the stark difference between the way we imagine the colon to lie within the abdomen and the way that it actually lies in most people. It is important to understand that if your colon does not look exactly like the one in our drawing, there is nothing wrong with you or your colon! Nonetheless, we describe the large bowel in this manner because these different segments of the colon really do exist (even if they do not position themselves exactly as we would like them to), and the description of the colon in this manner allows for easy communication between health care providers.

COLONIC SURGERY TERMINOLOGY

Patients with colonic disease often require surgery. There are many specific operations that can be performed on the colon, and you need to be familiar with the terminology so you know either what *has been done* or *will be done* surgically on a patient with colorectal disease.

- A colectomy refers to the surgical removal of the colon. In isolation, this may refer to the removal of the *entire* colon, but the term can be used to describe the removal of just a part of the colon as well:
  - A subtotal colectomy implies that the entire colon, with the exception of the rectum, is removed from the patient.
  - A total proctocolectomy implies that the entire colon, including the rectum, is removed from the patient.

- A right hemicolectomy refers to the removal of the ascending colon, possibly including the removal of the cecum and part or all of the transverse colon.
  - A right hemicolectomy also usually implies that an ileocolonic anastomosis has been created as well (if the cecum was removed during the surgery). This means that the ileum (the end of the small bowel) is sewn to the cut edge of the colon, so the bowel is now in continuity again. If an ileocolonic anastomosis is not created, the ileum may be brought out to the skin as an ileostomy (which connects to a drainage bag), and the distal remnant colon may either be oversewn (closed) or brought out to the skin via a colostomy (which connects to a separate drainage bag).
- A left hemicolectomy refers to the removal of the descending colon and possibly part or all of the transverse colon. A left hemicolectomy usually includes a colocolonic anastomosis whereby the proximal colon and the remnant left colon (the sigmoid and/or rectum) are directly sewn together so that the bowel is now in continuity again.
- Hartmann's procedure (also known as *Hartmann's operation* or *Hartmann's pouch*) refers to the removal of the rectosigmoid colon. This includes a colostomy (to drain the colon above the site of the resection) and closure of any remaining rectum.

COLITIS

Inflammation of the colon is referred to as *colitis*. There are many types of colitis, and you will encounter these commonly in clinical practice.

- **Ulcerative colitis (UC):** UC is a form of inflammatory bowel disease that primarily affects the large

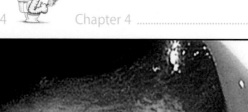

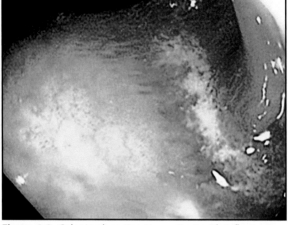

Figure 4-2. Colonic ulceration in a patient with inflammatory bowel disease and colitis.

bowel (although the terminal ileum can sometimes be affected via a process known as *backwash ileitis*) (Figure 4-2). UC typically involves the rectum and extends proximally. In some patients, only the left colon is involved, whereas other patients can have UC in their entire large bowel (known as *pancolitis*). In contrast to other forms of inflammatory bowel disease, such as Crohn's disease, UC is continuous in its involvement of the colon without interspersed areas of a normal large bowel. As with all inflammatory bowel disease, the exact cause of UC is not known. Although Crohn's disease classically produces transmural inflammation (which involves all layers of the bowel wall), UC results in primarily mucosal and submucosal inflammation and ulceration and not transmural inflammation.

Patients with UC typically have frequent watery bowel movements that are often bloody in nature. Patients with rectal involvement often experience a high degree of urgency (often with rectal spasms) and can develop incontinence. Some key points about UC include the following:

- UC is a chronic disease. Some patients will have a short period of disease followed by a long period of quiescence, whereas others will have a long and unremitting course of active colitis despite active therapy.

- UC puts patients at increased risk of developing colon cancer in their lifetime. Patients with UC need to undergo periodic screening to rule out dysplasia and/or cancer.

- Screening colonoscopy in patients with UC includes extensive biopsies from all segments of the colon to help rule out any dysplasia or cancer. Some people use the rule of 4 biopsies of each segment of the colon (eg, the cecum, ascending colon, hepatic flexure) to guide their biopsies, whereas others obtain 4 biopsies every 10 cm. This usually ends up meaning that patients have 32 to 36 biopsies obtained during colonoscopy. Any suspicious lesions or polyps should be biopsied or removed during colonoscopy. Patients who have high-grade dysplasia seen on their biopsies should be referred to a surgeon for consideration of colectomy. Patients with low-grade dysplasia can present a management dilemma; these patients can either undergo frequent surveillance or be referred for colectomy.

- There is no exact agreement on how often patients with UC should undergo screening/surveillance colonoscopy. The various

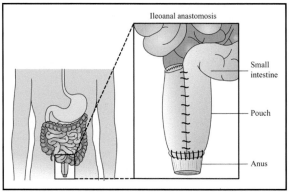

Figure 4-3. Ileoanal anastomosis following a colectomy.

gastrointestinal societies have all published different guidelines on this topic. Most would agree that patients with UC should begin screening colonoscopy after approximately 8 to 10 years of disease. Thereafter, patients undergo another colonoscopy every 1 to 3 years depending on the severity of their disease, symptoms, and findings on prior endoscopy.

○ In contrast to Crohn's disease (which has no cure), UC can be completely cured via colectomy. If there is no colon, there is no UC! A variety of surgical approaches are available to remove the colon in patients with UC. The most common approach is a proctocolectomy with an ileal pouch–anal anastomosis (Figure 4-3). This means that the entire colon is removed, and an artificial rectum (to serve as a vault or chamber for stool) is created using the terminal ileum. This artificial rectum is usually referred to as a *J pouch* because it is similar in shape to the letter J. Patients who undergo a proctocolectomy with the creation of a J pouch can either have a temporary ileostomy created (to allow the J pouch to heal before it is allowed to be placed in continuity with the remainder of the bowel), or they can go directly to using the J pouch without a diverting ileostomy above. Individual surgical practice varies in this regard.

○ Patients with UC who are not considered candidates for the creation of a J pouch usually undergo total colectomy with the creation of a permanent ileostomy. This is more commonly performed in patients who are elderly and/or obese.

○ Patients who have had their colon removed with the creation of a J pouch can still develop difficulties, most commonly pouchitis. Pouchitis can produce watery diarrhea, abdominal pain, and incontinence. Pouchitis can be infectious and an etiology or may be a manifestation of unsuspected Crohn's disease (ie, the patient had been previously misdiagnosed with UC but after colectomy developed signs/symptoms of Crohn's disease; see later). Infection with cytomegalovirus is a common cause of pouchitis after colectomy. Other viruses and bacteria can also contribute to pouchitis.

  • Some patients in whom there was strong evidence for UC will ultimately be found to have Crohn's disease. If these patients undergo proctocolectomy with pouch creation and Crohn's disease recurs within the pouch and cannot be controlled medically, the pouch must be removed. Patients in this situation often need to undergo creation of a permanent ileostomy.

- The bile duct disease primary sclerosing cholangitis is frequently seen in patients with colitis, especially UC. Although removing the colon does eliminate the disease of UC, it does not remove the risk of developing primary sclerosing cholangitis, and it does not modify the severity or progression of primary sclerosing cholangitis in patients who already have it.

- Medical therapy in patients with UC is similar to but different from that used in Crohn's disease (see Chapter 3 for more details on these medications). Corticosteroids, nonsteroidal immunosuppressive agents (eg, methotrexate, azathioprine, 6-MP), 5-aminosalicylic acid agents (eg, mesalamine), and biologic anti–tumor necrosis factor agents (eg, infliximab) are all used in patients with UC. Adalimumab and golimumab, both anti–tumor necrosis factor agents, and vedolizumab, an antiadhesion therapy, are also available for treating UC. The immunosuppressive agent cyclosporine is also occasionally used in patients with refractory UC. This agent is typically not used in patients with Crohn's disease and is often the drug of last resort before consideration of colectomy.

- The decision of whether or not to remove the colon in a patient with UC is often difficult and challenging. Obviously, if there is high-grade dysplasia or cancer seen on endoscopy, there is little to debate. If patients have poorly controlled colitis or are failing medical therapy, surgery is often the best option. Nonetheless, many patients are very hesitant to undergo colectomy. This is especially common in young patients because they worry about how an ileostomy (even a temporary one) would affect their personal life, including

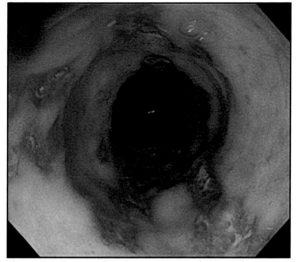

Figure 4-4. Severe colitis due to cytomegalovirus infection in a patient after renal transplantation.

their sexual life, and their ability to be physically, socially, and sexually active. Sometimes patients with severe colitis will attempt to delay or forestall colectomy for emotional rather than medical reasons.

  - UC can have extraintestinal manifestations just like Crohn's disease (see Chapter 3 for more on this).

- **Infectious colitis:** Infectious colitis, as the name implies, occurs when a microorganism (either bacterial, parasitic, or viral) infects the colon with resulting injury. Common bacterial causes of colitis include *Salmonella* and *Shigella*, *Escherichia coli*, and *Clostridium difficile*. Cytomegalovirus infection can also cause acute colitis, often in immunocompromised patients (Figure 4-4).

Some additional key points on infectious colitis include the following:

- *E coli* can produce typical inflammatory colitis or, in some patients infected with the 0157:H7 variant, a life-threatening enterohemorrhagic infection that is often associated with renal failure from so-called *hemolytic uremic syndrome*.

- *C difficile* colitis is commonly encountered among hospitalized patients and/or patients taking antibiotics. *C difficile* can produce fevers, high-volume watery diarrhea, and stereotypical pseudomembranes within the lumen of the colon. *C difficile* infection is also sometimes referred to as *pseudomembranous colitis* because of this fact. *C difficile* infection often occurs when the normal balance of microorganisms within the large bowel is disrupted and the *C difficile* organisms are allowed to reproduce unchecked. *C difficile* colitis may be very difficult to treat, and patients are prone to relapse. Most patients with *C difficile* colitis are treated with the antibiotics metronidazole or vancomycin.

- **Ischemic colitis:** Ischemic colitis occurs in the setting of an interruption in blood flow to the colon itself. Blood flow can be blocked due to vascular disease (atherosclerosis) or embolic disease (a clot forming in an artery that feeds the colon) or a vascular spasm that results in temporary blockage of blood flow. Ischemic colitis can also occur in the setting of a low-flow state without an actual obstruction (ie, hypotension from acute blood loss). Patients with ischemic colitis will often present with bloody diarrhea and abdominal pain that is crampy in nature. Patients will often have disproportionate pain in the setting of a relatively benign abdominal examination. Most patients with ischemic colitis will have mucosal and submucosal injury with hemorrhage and sloughing of the colonic lining. Surprisingly, most patients with ischemic colitis recover with conservative treatment (ie, fluid resuscitation, antibiotics). Patients who have transmural ischemia are at high risk for spontaneous perforation and are often treated surgically with partial or total colectomy. Most experienced endoscopists can tell the difference between mucosal/submucosal injury and full-thickness (transmural) ischemia with associated bowel wall necrosis. This information can help guide treatment in several ways; a high-quality colonoscopy in a patient with ischemic colitis can help decide if surgery is indicated or not. Furthermore, a colonoscopy in the setting of ischemic colitis can often define the extent of the injury (ie, does the ischemia affect the right colon, the left colon, or the entire large bowel), which can also affect the choice of operation for the patient.

- **Microscopic colitis/lymphocytic colitis/collagenous colitis:** These 3 terms can be thought of as all referring to a form of colitis that produces high-volume watery diarrhea in the setting of a colon that looks normal to the eye during colonoscopy, but when biopsies from the colon in these patients are examined under a microscope, they look abnormal. These 3 terms may all be different phases or faces of the same disease, or they may be different diseases; there is some controversy on this point. Microscopic colitis and lymphocytic colitis are remarkable for a lymphocytic infiltrate within the colonic mucosa itself. Collagenous colitis is so named because patients with this disease have increased collagen deposition within the lamina propria of the colonic mucosa as well as increased inflammatory cells/lymphocytes in their colonic mucosa. As I mentioned previously, there is ongoing debate about whether these 3 diseases are truly separate illnesses or if they are all different facets of the same underlying process (ie, does microscopic colitis become collagenous colitis over time?). These diseases are generally treated with anti-inflammatory agents (mesalamine or topical steroids), antidiarrheal agents, and bismuth-containing agents. The response to treatment is variable, with some patients having complete resolution of symptoms and others having intractable watery diarrhea for many years.

DIVERTICULOSIS AND DIVERTICULITIS

Diverticulosis refers to the presence of diverticula in the colon. Diverticula are pockets or outpouchings in the colonic wall (Figure 4-5). Diverticula can occur anywhere in the gastrointestinal tract, but they most commonly occur in the colon. In most patients, the presence of these diverticula (which can occur anywhere in the colon and can be quite numerous) are of no clinical consequence. Colonic diverticula are a common finding during colonoscopy. It should be noted that diverticula themselves are really pseudodiverticula in that they do not contain a full bowel wall. They are usually just composed of mucosa, submucosa, and sometimes muscularis propria. No one really knows what causes these diverticula; it may be genes, diet, or a combination of both.

Diverticula can cause trouble for patients in 2 ways: bleeding and infection. Diverticular bleeding is quite common. It usually presents as painless hematochezia (bright red blood per rectum) that can be high volume and lead to hypotension and so on. Endoscopy in these

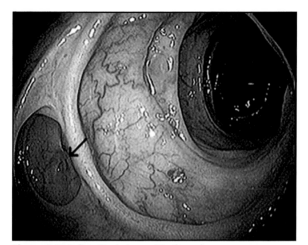

Figure 4-5. A diverticula (arrow) in the colon.

patients is often difficult because it can be quite a challenge to identify the actual bleeding diverticula in a patient who may have hundreds of diverticula, all of which may have some fresh and old blood in them. If the actual bleeding diverticula can be identified during colonoscopy, endoscopic approaches such as thermal therapy, injection therapy, and clip placement are all effective. If the actual bleeding diverticula cannot be identified, interventional radiology techniques such as angiography with embolization are often needed. If patients have recurrent episodes of bleeding, they sometimes undergo a partial colectomy to remove the area of the colon with the densest concentration of diverticula (but this does not reduce the risk of future bleeding from any of the remaining diverticula).

Diverticulitis refers to an infection of diverticula. Trapped stool can sometimes lead to these infections, and other times diverticula can become infected for unclear reasons. Patients with diverticulitis tend to have localized abdominal pain, fevers, chills, and other signs of systemic infection. Diverticulitis can range from mild (often treated on an outpatient basis with oral antibiotics) to severe (with abscess formation, perforation, and a need for urgent/emergent surgery). Diverticulitis is usually diagnosed via computed tomography (CT) scans or, less commonly, via colonoscopy (where it can occasionally mimic malignancy). There is little that can be done to prevent an episode of diverticulitis in patients with diverticulosis.

COLORECTAL CANCER

Colorectal cancer remains a major problem around the world. Fortunately, we live in an era where widespread information about colorectal cancer is available and effective screening tests exist.

Colon cancers are believed to arise from adenomatous polyps (Figure 4-6). Over time, these polyps undergo the so-called *adenoma-to-carcinoma sequence*. This term reflects a change in the histopathology of adenomatous polyps in the colon over time, with more ominous and aggressive features seen in more advanced polyps. In general, polyps progress from tubular adenomas to tubulovillous adenomas and from adenomas with low-grade dysplasia to those with high-grade dysplasia, carcinoma in situ (findings suggestive of localized early cancer), and, ultimately, adenocarcinoma (full-blown colorectal cancer). Because colorectal cancers arise from polyps, an enormous effort has been undertaken around the world to promote screening examinations to detect precancerous polyps and remove them before they can turn into cancer. Screening examinations also have the ability to detect colorectal cancers before they metastasize to other organs.

Most colorectal cancers occur in patients with no increased risk or family history of the disease. These tumors

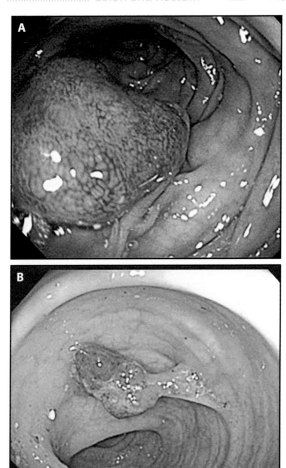

Figure 4-6. (A) A sessile colon polyp. (B) A pedunculated colon polyp and its stalk.

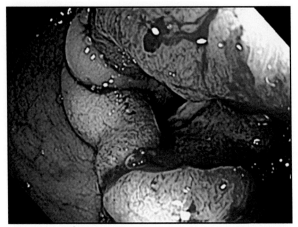

Figure 4-7. Sporadic colon cancer discovered during screening colonoscopy in an asymptomatic patient.

are referred to as *sporadic cancers* (Figure 4-7). Patients with a family history of colorectal cancer (especially in first-degree relatives) as well as patients with polyposis syndromes (eg, familial adenomatous polyposis and hereditary nonpolyposis colorectal cancer, among others) are at increased lifetime risk of developing colorectal (and other forms of) cancer and require special surveillance protocols. Patients with inflammatory bowel disease with colitis (either UC or Crohn's disease) are also at increased risk for developing colorectal cancer and require special screening protocols.

As a general rule, average-risk individuals should begin colorectal cancer screening at 50 years old. There is evidence that African Americans of average risk should undergo their first screening examination at 45 years old. A variety of screening tests are available, including the following:

- Colonoscopy is the most widely used colorectal cancer screening test in the Western world.

Colonoscopy has many advantages; it allows direct visualization of the entire colon real-time in full color and often in high-definition/high-resolution images. Colonoscopy is not just diagnostic but is also a therapeutic modality because any polyps seen during colonoscopy can either be completely removed or at the very least biopsied. Recommendations for future screening can be made based on the results obtained during colonoscopy and based on the pathologic subtype of any polyps found. Colonoscopy is the most invasive colorectal cancer screening test and does carry risks of sedation, perforation, bleeding, etc. Colonoscopy also requires a formal bowel preparation (which often involves drinking up to a gallon of a solution designed to flush any and all stool out of the colon), which many patients find unpleasant. If a colonoscopy in an average-risk patient is completely normal, most patients will undergo their next colonoscopy in 10 years. If polyps are identified, the interval to the next colonoscopy is determined based on the number, size, type, and location of the polyps.

- Flexible sigmoidoscopy is an endoscopic procedure similar to a colonoscopy; however, instead of using a colonoscope, flexible sigmoidoscopy uses a shorter endoscope (known as a *sigmoidoscope*) that is only able to evaluate the left colon. Flexible sigmoidoscopy does not evaluate the entire colon but has nonetheless been shown to detect polyps and reduce mortality from colorectal cancer. Flexible sigmoidoscopy was once widely performed but has largely been supplanted by colonoscopy. An old joke about flexible sigmoidoscopy is that it is analogous to performing mammography on only one breast; fully half of the colon (or more) goes completely unvisualized during flexible sigmoidoscopy.

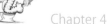
Any polyps or cancers above the level that the sigmoidoscope can reach will go undetected. Flexible sigmoidoscopy also requires some sort of bowel preparation (either drinking a solution to flush the colon of stool or enemas) and can be performed with or without sedation. Flexible sigmoidoscopy, like colonoscopy, also carries a risk of perforation and bleeding. If the flexible sigmoidoscopy is completely normal, for an average-risk patient, it is recommended that patients undergo their next flexible sigmoidoscopy in 5 years. As with colonoscopy, the identification of polyps during a flexible sigmoidoscopy may prompt a shorter interval between flexible sigmoidoscopies or undergoing a full colonoscopy.

- CT colonoscopy (also known as *CT colonography* or *virtual colonoscopy*) refers to looking at the large bowel using a CT scanner that is able to create high-resolution images of the entire colon. Modern CT colonoscopy protocols allow for the detection of polyps or tumors in the colon. Some CT colonoscopy protocols create 3-dimensional images and allow the viewer to "fly through" the colon and see a view very similar to what one would see during actual colonoscopy. Advantages of CT colonography include the fact it is noninvasive in nature and can detect larger polyps and cancers. Disadvantages of this technique include the following: patients still typically need to undergo a formal bowel preparation; patients are exposed to radiation; the test may not be as good as endoscopy at identifying small polyps; and if any lesion is seen on a CT scan, the patient must then undergo a regular colonoscopy. If there is not an endoscopist ready and waiting on the day of the CT scan (which is generally the case), the patient has to come back a different day for colonoscopy and thus must undergo 2 bowel preparations.

- Fecal occult blood testing (also known as *guaiac testing*) looks for microscopic traces of blood in the stool. These tests are based on the idea that colon cancers and possibly large polyps may occasionally bleed and that their presence could be detected by looking for small amounts of blood in the stool. These tests are very inexpensive; a small card is given to a patient, and the patient puts a small sample of stool onto the card. If there is blood in the stool, a color change will be visible on the card when it is exposed to certain chemicals. Fecal occult blood testing was once widely used as a colorectal cancer screening test for the following reasons: the test is cheap, safe, and carries virtually no risks, and fecal occult blood testing has been shown to reduce the risk of death from colorectal cancer. Fecal occult blood as an isolated test is less commonly performed in the current era given the widespread use of colonoscopy.

- Fecal DNA testing, although not actively used in most colorectal cancer screening programs, is worthy of brief mention. The idea behind this test is that your colon and any colon cancers will periodically shed cells into the lumen of the bowel, which pass with stool. These cancer cells should contain abnormal DNA sequences, which can be tested for. The idea goes even further in that tumors of the lung (which may produce coughing and then swallowing of shed tumor cells), esophagus, stomach, and small bowel may also shed cells into the gastrointestinal tract. Thus, fecal DNA testing may potentially detect many forms of aerodigestive cancer.

- Kits that test for both fecal occult blood and evaluate fecal DNA are now widely available. The advantages of these tests are that they are noninvasive and give a lot of information to patients and health care providers. A positive test still warrants a colonoscopy.

ANORECTAL WOES

Gastroenterology encompasses the diagnosis and management of a variety of diseases of the anus and rectum. Although these do not exactly qualify as party talk, these diseases are important to know and understand because patients who have anorectal troubles are often in great distress and in need of significant help.

- Hemorrhoids are a common complaint. When patients say "I have hemorrhoids" (and they say it all the time!), what they really mean is that they have dilated and/or inflamed blood vessels around their anus. Every human being on earth has these blood vessels around their anus; we only describe them as hemorrhoids when they become symptomatic or troublesome. Sometimes hemorrhoids can simply be a nuisance; they make cleaning up after a bowel movement more labor intensive. Hemorrhoids can become inflamed and/or thrombosed (have a blood clot inside of them), which can lead to acute anal pain. Hemorrhoids can also bleed, and the blood loss in some patients can be significant. Hemorrhoids can be external (visible to the naked eye or palpable with a finger when wiping) or internal. Internal hemorrhoids are best seen during endoscopy when the endoscope is bent back on itself to view the distal rectum (known as *endoscopic retroflexion*). Hemorrhoids can become symptomatic if a patient strains against a hard bowel movement, has prolonged periods of sitting, etc. If hemorrhoids simply become inflamed periodically, patients can often get by via taking stool softeners and/or using over-the-counter topical steroid creams to reduce inflammation. If hemorrhoids bleed, become thrombosed, or become a chronic source of pain and discomfort, many patients opt to have their hemorrhoids treated in a more definitive manner. Hemorrhoids can be removed surgically, ligated with sutures or rubber bands, injected with sclerosing agents (that promote clot formation and scarring of the hemorrhoid), or treated with thermal therapies (that also aim to promote clot formation). Some of these procedures (banding, sclerotherapy, and thermal therapy) can be performed with an endoscope or other specialized devices. Most modern hemorrhoid therapies can be performed on an outpatient basis, which is very different than it was in the past when the mainstay of treatment was surgery.

- Anal warts are a sexually transmitted disease and a manifestation of the human papilloma virus. Sometimes patients will mistake anal warts for hemorrhoids and vice versa. A variety of topical medications can be used to treat these warts. Other therapies, including cryoablation and thermal therapies like cauterization, are available. Large warts may have to be excised surgically. In practice, anal warts are very difficult to cure, and many patients have ongoing disease despite aggressive therapy. The vaccine currently available against the human papilloma virus should protect against these types of warts.

- Anal cancer is a form of squamous cell carcinoma. Most anal cancers are probably also related to human papilloma virus infection, which is usually spread through sexual activity. Anal cancers are more commonly seen in patients with HIV or other forms of immunosuppression, as well as in those patients who have chronic anal inflammation (patients with inflammatory bowel disease). Smoking appears to be a risk factor as well. Some patients will mistake early anal cancer for hemorrhoids, resulting in a delay in diagnosis.

- Anal fissures are considered a break in the skin overlying the anus. Patients can experience excruciating pain from anal fissures, especially during a bowel movement or periods of prolonged sitting. The fissure itself may be quite small despite the severity of discomfort. The exact cause of anal fissures is debatable but may be related to straining during defecation. Many anal fissures will spontaneously heal or may require medical treatment with stool softeners or topical agents to relax the anal sphincter muscles (which is thought to promote healing). Topical agents that can be used include nitroglycerin and calcium channel blockers. If fissures do not respond to medical therapy, surgery can be undertaken, although this carries a risk of sphincter injury and subsequent incontinence.

- Anal fistulas are defined as a communication between the anal canal and the perianal skin. Anal fistulas are a source of significant morbidity. Anal fistulas can give rise to perianal abscesses, which require aggressive drainage. Anal fistulas are more commonly seen in patients with Crohn's disease. Anal fistulas may be multifocal and can trace a tortuous path from within the anal canal, through the soft tissues of the perineum and buttocks, and out through the skin. The rise of biologic agents to treat patients in Crohn's disease (eg, infliximab) has been a major advancement in the treatment of anal fistulas as well as other forms of fistulas seen in Crohn's disease, including fistulas between bowel loops (enteroenteric fistulas) or the bowel to the skin (enterocutaneous fistulas). Many anal fistulas ultimately require surgical treatment. Surgical treatments are generally aimed at promoting drainage of the fistula, eliminating any abscesses, and promoting healing of the fistula, and they should be undertaken while

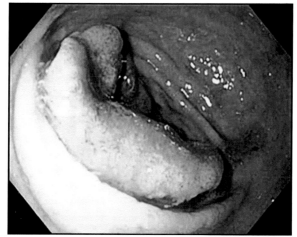

Figure 4-8. A large rectal cancer.

simultaneously treating any underlying causes of the fistula (eg, Crohn's disease).

- Rectal cancer, although closely related to colon cancer, is treated somewhat differently and merits some special discussion. Most colon cancers (if not metastatic) can be treated by local excision and a colocolonic anastomosis. Rectal cancers, defined as adenocarcinomas that occur in the distal 12 to 15 cm of the large bowel, are technically more difficult to operate on given their location deep within the pelvis (Figure 4-8). It can be harder for a surgeon to remove all of the cancer in some of these patients. Rectal cancers also present a special challenge because their resection may also include removal of the anal sphincter complex; such patients typically undergo the creation of a colostomy. Special surgical techniques (ie, total mesorectal excision) have been

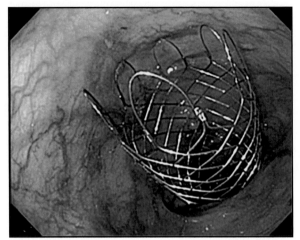

Figure 4-9. A self-expanding metal stent placed across an obstructing colorectal cancer to reestablish bowel patency.

developed to provide better outcomes in patients undergoing surgery for rectal cancer. Early rectal cancers (defined as tumors that have not spread to the deep layers of the bowel wall, lymph nodes, or other organs) can undergo simple transanal resection. Unfortunately, these are the least commonly encountered rectal cancers. Most rectal cancers are found in what is referred to as a locally advanced state; these tumors invade to deep layers of the bowel wall or completely obliterate the bowel wall and often have local nodal spread. Most patients with locally advanced rectal cancer

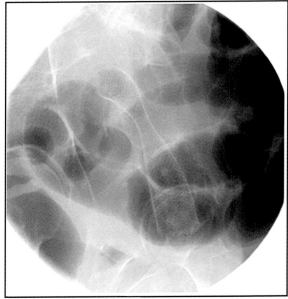

Figure 4-10. An x-ray image of a self-expanding stent in the colon after placement to treat a malignant obstructing colorectal cancer.

need to undergo neoadjuvant therapy via chemoradiation before surgery is attempted. Patients may develop bowel obstruction from rectal cancer. These patients can be treated with a stent while undergoing chemoradiation therapy to relieve symptoms of obstruction (Figures 4-9 and 4-10).

BIBLIOGRAPHY

Adler DG, Young-Fadok TM, Smyrk T, Garces YI, Baron TH. Preoperative chemoradiation therapy after placement of a self-expanding metal stent in a patient with an obstructing rectal cancer: clinical and pathologic findings. *Gastrointest Endosc.* 2002;55(3):435-437.

Atkin WS, Edwards R, Kralj-Hans I, et al; UK Flexible Sigmoidoscopy Trial Investigators. Once-only flexible sigmoidoscopy screening in prevention of colorectal cancer: a multicentre randomised controlled trial. *Lancet.* 2010;375(9726):1624-1633.

Brandt LJ, Boley SJ. AGA technical review on intestinal ischemia. American Gastrointestinal Association. *Gastroenterology.* 2000;118(5):954-968.

Feurer ME, Hilden K, Adler DG. Primary sclerosing cholangitis and distribution of inflammatory bowel disease. *Clin Gastroenterol Hepatol.* 2012;10(12):1418; author reply 1418-1419.

Levin B, Lieberman DA, McFarland B, et al; American Cancer Society Colorectal Cancer Advisory Group; US Multi-Society Task Force; American College of Radiology Colon Cancer Committee. Screening and surveillance for the early detection of colorectal cancer and adenomatous polyps, 2008: a joint guideline from the American Cancer Society, the US Multi-Society Task Force on Colorectal Cancer, and the American College of Radiology. *CA Cancer J Clin.* 2008;58(3):130-160.

Moore J, Jones K, Adler DG. Management of rectal cancer. *Commun Oncol.* 2009;6:265-270.

Moore J, Jones K, Adler DG. Preoperative evaluation of rectal cancer: evaluation, diagnosis, and staging. *Commun Oncol.* 2009;6:161-165.

Yen EF, Pardi DS. Review of the microscopic colitides. *Curr Gastroenterol Rep.* 2011;13(5):458-464.

Chapter 5

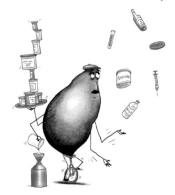

Liver

The liver, like the pancreas, is poorly understood by the general population. Most people have an understanding of what their esophagus and stomach do just from their day-to-day life, but the liver remains largely a mystery. Most patients know that drinking causes cirrhosis (even if they do not really understand what cirrhosis really is) and are aware that some people get liver transplantation, but that is usually about it.

In reality, the liver is a fascinating organ that performs a great number of functions, all of which are necessary for normal health and digestive function. This chapter will review the basics of liver anatomy, physiology, and a variety of disease states of the liver that you will encounter when treating patients.

Adler DG. *The Little GI Book: An Easily Digestible Guide to Understanding Gastroenterology, Second Edition* (pp 127-160).

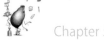
ANATOMY

The liver is a wedge-shaped organ that sits in the right upper quadrant of the abdomen. The dome of the liver sits just below the diaphragm, and the right margin of the liver abuts the ribs on the right side. The underside of the liver abuts the right kidney, the colon, and the duodenum. The left lobe of the liver often drapes across the anterior wall of the stomach.

The liver is classically divided into the right and left hepatic lobes with 2 smaller hepatic lobes sandwiched in between. These are referred to as the *caudate lobe* and the *quadrate lobe*. The caudate lobe is superior, whereas the quadrate lobe is inferior anatomically.

Vascular Anatomy

Blood flows into the liver from several sources. The portal vein carries blood into the liver that has already drained from the small bowel, large bowel, pancreas, gall-bladder, and spleen. The liver receives most of its blood via the portal vein. The liver also receives arterial blood from the hepatic artery. The hepatic artery is a branch of the celiac artery, which is the first major artery to branch off of the aorta below the level of the diaphragm.

Blood flows through the liver, where it is processed in a variety of manners, ultimately passing through the small sinusoidal vessels. Blood is then pooled into the central veins of each hepatic lobule, which ultimately form the large hepatic veins. These veins drain blood into the inferior vena cava, which ultimately returns blood to the right side of the heart.

Biliary Anatomy

We will cover the bile ducts more extensively in Chapter 6, but it is important to know at this stage of the game that the liver makes bile (which is useful for helping to digest fat, among other reasons) and secretes the bile into microscopic canaliculi and then into tiny intrahepatic ducts. These intrahepatic ducts join ever larger ducts and ultimately form the large extrahepatic bile ducts that carry bile to the duodenum, where it mixes with food during digestion. The extrahepatic ducts consist of the right and left hepatic ducts, which join to form the common hepatic duct. The common hepatic duct drains into the common bile duct, which drains into the small bowel. The gallbladder is connected to the common bile duct via the cystic duct. The cystic duct is often shaped like an old-fashioned telephone cord (for those of us who actually remember that phones used to have cords that connected them to the wall).

Microscopic Anatomy

The liver is mostly made up of cells referred to as *hepatocytes*. The hepatocytes do much of the day-to-day work of the liver as described later. Hepatocytes are organized into structures known as *portal tracts*. These portal tracts are generally thought to contain a hepatic artery branch, the portal vein branch, and a small bile duct. In this manner, blood is processed, and bile is manufactured and secreted. The liver also contains a variety of other cell types, including macrophages (known as *Kupffer cells*), connective tissue cells, stellate cells (which mediate the formation of fibrosis in the liver), and endothelial and sinusoidal cells (which line microscopic blood vessels in the liver).

FUNCTIONS OF THE LIVER

As a medical student, I was amazed by the number and type of functions that the liver was able to perform. There is really no other comparable organ to the liver in terms of diversity of function. Patients with acute liver injury can often become critically ill within hours; this is a testament to the vital nature of the liver and all it does. The following is a summary of some of the key functions of the liver.

Synthetic Functions

The liver manufactures a variety of substances necessary for normal health and function. Some substances that the liver produces include the following:

- Coagulation factors that allow normal blood clotting to occur
- Cholesterol and triglycerides
- Amino acids (necessary for protein synthesis)
- Bile
- Glucose (via a process known as *gluconeogenesis*)
- Glycogen (a form of starch that serves as a long-term storage form of glucose); it is worth noting that other organs can make glycogen as well
- Albumin (the major protein in the blood)
- Angiotensin (a hormone that helps raise blood pressure)

Detoxification/Catabolism

The liver plays a major role in breaking down many substances in the bloodstream and in detoxifying the blood as well. Some examples include the following:

- Drug metabolism and detoxification (this allows potentially harmful molecules to be excreted from the body via urine or bile)
- Hormone degradation (to help allow for proper hormone levels and balance)
- Ammonia degradation (which is converted into urea for removal from the body via the kidneys)

Storage

The liver is a storage site for the following:
- Iron
- Copper
- Vitamin A
- Vitamin D
- Vitamin B$_{12}$

CIRRHOSIS

We should discuss cirrhosis early in this chapter because a working knowledge of cirrhosis is important for understanding almost all the liver diseases that follow. Just as chronic pancreatitis implies permanent scarring to the pancreas, cirrhosis implies permanent scarring of the liver known as *fibrosis*. Cirrhosis is the final end result of a variety of hepatic disease processes. As the liver becomes progressively fibrotic and scarred, it develops a structure of abnormal fibrotic nodules and gradually loses function. Many patients with mild cirrhosis may have few outward signs of liver disease. Patients with advanced or decompensated cirrhosis may be profoundly ill and debilitated by their disease, and many patients succumb to cirrhosis and its complications.

Understanding portal hypertension is critical to truly understanding cirrhosis. As a liver becomes progressively more diseased and fibrotic, blood flowing into the liver via the portal vein meets increasing resistance to flow (ie, the fibrotic cirrhotic liver is not as receptive to portal blood flow as a normal liver) and pressure in the portal vein, and the vessels that flow into it rise. Patients with cirrhosis are also referred to as hyperdynamic with regard to their circulation; they tend to have a low blood pressure state in the setting of an increased

cardiac output. This combination of a fibrotic liver and portal hypertension leads to many of the complications of cirrhosis, including gastrointestinal bleeding, ascites, peritonitis, renal dysfunction, and encephalopathy.

You have probably seen many patients with cirrhosis in your day-to-day life and not realized it. Patients with cirrhosis often have telltale physical findings that belie their underlying cirrhotic state. Contrary to popular belief, many patients with cirrhosis do not have jaundice (although some do). Reddening of the palms (known as *palmar erythema*), so-called *spider veins* (angiomata) on the face and chest (prominent superficial blood vessels in the skin that look somewhat like spiders), abnormal fluid collection within the abdomen (known as *ascites*), an enlarged spleen (known as *hypersplenism*), swelling of the lower extremities, easy bruising (from deficient vitamin K–dependent clotting factors synthesis in the liver), and gynecomastia are all commonly seen in patients with cirrhosis. Once you learn to look for the signs of cirrhosis on physical examination, they are generally easy to spot, and you may find yourself noticing them in individuals you meet outside of the hospital as well!

Ascites

The term *ascites* refers to the abnormal collection of fluid within the abdomen. Most patients with ascites have underlying cirrhosis and portal hypertension, although ascites can be caused by other diseases. Patients with liver disease who develop cirrhosis often have so-called *shifting dullness* (increased girth in their abdomen due to fluid accumulation that moves when the patient changes positions or is examined with palpation) and lower extremity edema (swelling). The fluid accumulates in the abdominal cavity due to a combination of low serum albumin (which is produced in limited quantities by the cirrhotic liver and which ordinarily promotes fluid retention in the vascular space) and portal hypertension, which promotes the migration of fluid out of venous structures and into surrounding tissues.

Ascites is usually easy to detect on physical examination and with imaging studies. An abdominal ultrasound, computed tomography (CT) scan, or magnetic resonance imaging (MRI) are all viable ways to detect ascites, although right quadrant ultrasound is typically chosen first because it is the easiest test to do and the least expensive.

If ascites is seen during a right quadrant ultrasound, it can be aspirated using a needle via a procedure known as *paracentesis*. Paracentesis can be either diagnostic or therapeutic.

Diagnostic paracentesis typically only involves the removal of 10 to 50 mL of fluid. This fluid can then be sent for analysis to help determine the type of ascites that is present and whether or not there are signs of infection in the fluid. As I mentioned earlier, although most ascites occur due to cirrhosis, other causes, including cancer, heart failure, and tuberculosis, can also lead to ascites. An analysis of the ascitic fluid can help determine the etiology of the ascites itself. Analysis involves cytologic evaluation (to look for cancer or signs of tuberculosis), culture to look for the type and severity of bacterial infection, a white blood cell count (also elevated in patients with ascetic fluid infection), and measurement of total protein and albumin level in the fluid.

It is always worth measuring the serum-ascites albumin gradient (SAAG) on aspirated ascitic fluid. The SAAG is easily calculated by subtracting the concentration of albumin in ascitic fluid from the concentration of albumin in the serum. An SAAG that is greater than 1.1 g/dL in the setting of a low total protein level in the ascitic fluid strongly suggests that the ascites is due to cirrhosis.

Patients with ascites are at high risk for developing spontaneous infection of the ascetic fluid known as *spontaneous bacterial peritonitis* (SBP). If the fluid analysis shows a neutrophil count greater than 250/mm^3, the patient is presumed to have SBP. SBP is treated with antibiotics, and patients typically improve rapidly, although recurrent infections are common and some patients require chronic antibiotic use.

In contrast to diagnostic paracentesis, large-volume paracentesis is performed when patients accumulate very large amounts of ascitic fluid in their abdomen that cannot be controlled by approaches including dietary sodium restriction and diuretics, such as furosemide and spironolactone. It is not uncommon for patients to accumulate many liters of ascitic fluid within their abdominal cavity. This fluid puts patients at risk for SBP, can compromise their ability to breathe easily due to limited diaphragmatic excursion, and can be painful (a condition known as *tense ascites*). When performing large-volume paracentesis, the fluid must be withdrawn slowly to avoid rapid fluid shifts, and patients should receive concurrent intravenous albumin infusion. If the fluid is removed too quickly, patients can become hypotensive and require resuscitation.

Patients with uncontrollable ascites who require frequent large-volume paracentesis may benefit from a transjugular intrahepatic portosystemic shunt (TIPS). A TIPS procedure involves the creation of a shunt between the inflowing portal vein and the outflowing hepatic vein via the use of a vascular stent that is placed by an interventional radiologist through an access point in the jugular vein. The TIPS serves to lower portal venous pressure and promotes blood flow through the liver with a reduction in overall vascular resistance.

Bleeding

In Chapter 1, we discussed esophageal variceal bleeding in some detail. To review briefly, portal hypertension commonly leads to the formation of varices in the esophagus (due to high portal vein pressure that is transmitted to esophageal venous structures, which when engorged with blood become known as *varices*), although varices can occur in the stomach, small bowel, and rectum as well. These varices, especially esophageal and gastric varices, are at high risk for spontaneous hemorrhage. Esophageal varices are often treated to good effect via esophageal variceal banding and/or sclerotherapy. Gastric varices respond poorly to these techniques, and when gastric variceal bleeding occurs, it is often massive and life threatening. Bleeding from varices in other locations is uncommon but can occur. Uncontrollable variceal bleeding is often treated via TIPS in an effort to reduce the portal venous pressure and decompress the bleeding varices. Endoscopic banding can also be performed to stop gastric varices from bleeding, but it is usually used as a stopgap measure until a TIPS can be performed (Figure 5-1).

Hepatic Encephalopathy

Hepatic encephalopathy refers to the clinical findings of confusion and/or an altered mental status that is commonly seen in patients with cirrhosis. Hepatic encephalopathy can be mild, moderate, or severe in nature, and mild encephalopathy may be difficult to detect clinically. Patients with mild hepatic encephalopathy may have difficulty sleeping or altered sleep/wake patterns (often sleeping during the day and being awake at night), irritability, forgetfulness, mild confusion, and poor concentration. As encephalopathy progresses, patients may become somnolent, frankly confused, and disoriented. Severe encephalopathy can lead to unconsciousness and coma, culminating in death if not treated. Patients with hepatic encephalopathy often develop a characteristic flapping motion in their hands and arms that can be seen on formal testing known as *asterixis*.

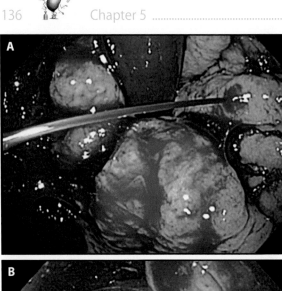

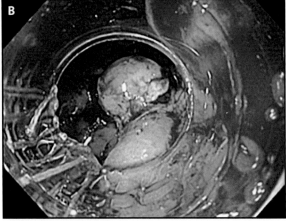

Figure 5-1. (A) Actively bleeding gastric varices in a patient with alcoholic cirrhosis. (B) The same patient as in A after band ligation with hemostasis.

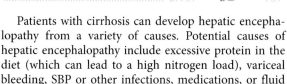
Patients with cirrhosis can develop hepatic encephalopathy from a variety of causes. Potential causes of hepatic encephalopathy include excessive protein in the diet (which can lead to a high nitrogen load), variceal bleeding, SBP or other infections, medications, or fluid and electrolyte imbalances.

It is believed that high circulating levels of ammonia may play a role in the development of hepatic encephalopathy. Treatment is aimed at identifying and addressing underlying causes (eg, gastrointestinal bleeding, SBP) and taking steps to reduce serum ammonia levels (although actual ammonia levels correlate poorly with the presence or severity of hepatic encephalopathy). Agents that reduce ammonia production or absorption are often used to treat hepatic encephalopathy. These include the antibiotics neomycin and rifaximin (to kill bacteria living in the bowel that generate ammonia) and the disaccharide lactulose (which converts ammonia in the gut to nonabsorbable ammonium). Of note, lactulose produces significant diarrhea. Patients with hepatic encephalopathy are typically instructed to titrate their dose of lactulose to a goal of 3 to 5 bowel movements per day. Lactulose has a very sweet taste that some patients find difficult to tolerate.

HEREDITARY LIVER DISEASES

There are many hereditary liver diseases that you will encounter in clinical practice. These can be thought of as inborn errors of metabolism that can affect the liver and other organs in many ways. Some of these diseases may manifest in childhood, whereas others will only manifest later in life. It is important to understand the key hereditary liver disorders because their recognition allows for proper treatment, and many of these patients are candidates for liver transplantation, which is often curative.

Some of the most common hereditary liver disorders are as follows.

Hereditary Hemochromatosis

The term *hereditary hemochromatosis* is used to describe disorders of hepatic iron metabolism. Patients with hemochromatosis store excess iron in their liver and other tissues and develop "iron overload." There are a variety of genetic abnormalities that can give rise to hemochromatosis. It takes many years to develop true iron overload; most patients with classic hemochromatosis (due to abnormalities in the *HFE* gene) present as adults with findings of cirrhosis and other symptoms of the disease. There is a juvenile form of the disease that can affect teenagers or people in their 20s as well.

Patients with hemochromatosis deposit iron into their liver to an extreme extent. The iron accumulates in hepatocytes directly as well as in cells known as *macrophages*. Iron deposition of the liver can lead directly to inflammation and cirrhosis. Patients with hemochromatosis are at high risk of developing hepatocellular cancer (HCC). Iron also accumulates secondarily in other tissues, including the pancreas (resulting in diabetes), the skin (which gives patients an unusual pigmentation that can look gray or brown), the pituitary gland (which can lead to sexual dysfunction, amenorrhea, delayed or impaired puberty, and other hormonal disturbances), and the heart (which can lead to cardiomyopathy, or arrhythmia). The combination of the unusual skin pigmentation and diabetes in patients with hemochromatosis has given rise to the term *bronze diabetes*.

If patients with hemochromatosis are recognized early in the course of their disease (either through genetic testing due to a relative with known disease or through recognition of abnormally high iron indices), patients can undergo phlebotomy to remove iron-rich red blood cells from their system as a means of producing iron depletion.

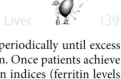
Patients donate 1 unit of blood periodically until excess iron is removed from their system. Once patients achieve normal iron levels in normal iron indices (ferritin levels and transferrin levels), they can undergo phlebotomy less frequently but still need to do this periodically because the underlying genetic defect is still present; these patients will simply start accumulating iron again if phlebotomy is not continued.

I should emphasize that the risk of HCC is very high in these patients; even successful phlebotomy does not fully eliminate the risk of developing liver cancer. These patients need to be monitored closely by periodic imaging studies to ensure they do not develop HCC. If HCC is detected or if phlebotomy is insufficient to treat the iron overload, patients should be referred for evaluation for liver transplantation. Family members of patients with hereditary hemochromatosis should be appropriately screened at a young age. Identification of the disease early in life (with appropriate phlebotomy) can prevent the development of iron-mediated injury to the liver or other organs.

Alpha-1 Antitrypsin Deficiency

Alpha-1 antitrypsin deficiency is another inherited disorder of liver metabolism. Alpha-1 antitrypsin inhibits the function of certain proteases (enzymes that help degrade protein). In patients with alpha-1 antitrypsin deficiency, there is a genetic error that leads to the production of an abnormal and inactive form of alpha-1 antitrypsin. This abnormal form of alpha-1 antitrypsin is both nonfunctional and abnormally accumulated in the liver itself. As alpha-1 antitrypsin accumulates within hepatocytes, liver dysfunction occurs. Patients with alpha-1 antitrypsin deficiency are also prone to lung disease, most commonly emphysema. Patients with alpha-1 antitrypsin deficiency tend to have a low serum alpha-1 antitrypsin level (because the molecule cannot effectively escape the liver to enter the bloodstream).

Patients with alpha-1 antitrypsin deficiency may present during the neonatal period with signs of jaundice and/or hepatitis. Other patients may not develop signs of liver disease, including cirrhosis, until they are teenagers. The majority of patients are recognized as adults, who often have cirrhosis at the time of diagnosis. These patients, like patients with hemochromatosis, are at risk for developing HCC. Patients with alpha-1 antitrypsin deficiency can develop liver disease, lung disease, or both.

The classic treatment for alpha-1 antitrypsin deficiency is liver transplantation. Once patients undergo liver transplantation, they no longer have the disease (ie, the new liver has normal alpha-1 antitrypsin production and does not go on to develop cirrhosis). Pre-existing lung disease does not resolve after liver transplantation.

Simple blood tests can give critically important information regarding the alpha-1 antitrypsin genotype. Normal individuals will have M alleles. Abnormal alpha-1 antitrypsin alleles are described as S or Z. Patients with a ZZ genotype have the most profound disease, although alpha-1 antitrypsin deficiency can develop in patients with SZ or SS genotypes. Most patients with the MZ genotype are asymptomatic.

Wilson's Disease

Wilson's disease refers to a genetic disorder in which copper excretion is impaired and copper deposits build up in the hepatocytes themselves. Wilson's disease is to copper what hemochromatosis is to iron; these are both disorders of abnormal metal accumulation in the liver. Patients with Wilson's disease have an abnormal copper-transporting enzyme that is coded for by a gene known as ATP7B. Patients with Wilson's disease have low levels of a copper-binding protein known as *ceruloplasmin*. Patients with Wilson's disease tend to have high urinary copper levels and low serum ceruloplasmin levels. Copper accumulates in the liver and causes direct

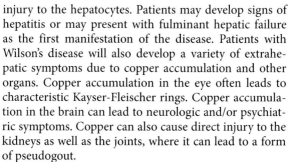
injury to the hepatocytes. Patients may develop signs of hepatitis or may present with fulminant hepatic failure as the first manifestation of the disease. Patients with Wilson's disease will also develop a variety of extrahepatic symptoms due to copper accumulation and other organs. Copper accumulation in the eye often leads to characteristic Kayser-Fleischer rings. Copper accumulation in the brain can lead to neurologic and/or psychiatric symptoms. Copper can also cause direct injury to the kidneys as well as the joints, where it can lead to a form of pseudogout.

If the disease is identified before hepatic failure develops, patients are often treated via chelation therapy. Chelators are oral agents that can directly bind copper and are then removed from the body via urinary excretion. The most commonly used chelating agents are d-penicillamine and trientine. Orally administered zinc can also reduce systemic copper levels. Patients are typically advised to avoid copper-rich foods such as liver, oysters, sun-dried tomatoes, certain nuts and seeds, and certain herbs. If the disease presents as fulminant hepatic failure, patients should undergo liver transplantation.

Hereditary Hyperbilirubinemia

The term *hereditary hyperbilirubinemia* refers to disorders of bilirubin metabolism. These may manifest shortly after birth or may not become clinically apparent until adulthood. Some of these disorders are of little clinical significance, whereas others are life threatening and require liver transplantation.

The classic disorder of bilirubin metabolism is known as *Gilbert's syndrome*. You probably know somebody with Gilbert's syndrome. Patients with Gilbert's syndrome have a genetic defect that produces an error in an enzyme known as *uridine 5'-diphospho-glucuronosyltransferase*. This enzyme is critical for normal bilirubin metabolism. Patients with Gilbert's syndrome develop what is known as an *unconjugated hyperbilirubinemia*. Specifically, these patients develop a mild form of jaundice during periods of metabolic stress (eg, illness, physical exertion, periods of poor sleep). These patients have a mildly elevated total serum bilirubin level, but almost none of the bilirubin will be conjugated. Conjugation refers to the process by which bilirubin is modified by the liver for excretion out of the body. Patients with Gilbert's syndrome will have periodic episodes of jaundice that are self-limited and resolve when the underlying problem goes away. The classic clinical presentation of Gilbert's syndrome is in a young person (often a student) who notices that he becomes jaundice during a stressful period such as finals week (during which time he has been eating badly, sleeping poorly due to pulling all-nighters, and has caught a cold!).

Crigler-Najjar syndrome is a more serious disorder of bilirubin metabolism. These patients have a more severe abnormality in the same gene that causes Gilbert's syndrome. Patients with Crigler-Najjar syndrome often develop unconjugated hyperbilirubinemia shortly after birth that can be severe. The hyperbilirubinemia can lead to a brain disturbance known as *kernicterus*. Patients with Crigler-Najjar syndrome often require liver transplantation at a young age.

In contrast, Dubin-Johnson syndrome produces a conjugated hyperbilirubinemia due to a genetic defect that leads to abnormal bile processing by the liver. Patients with Dubin-Johnson syndrome tend to do well over the long term because they have preserved liver function despite the disorder.

ACQUIRED LIVER DISEASES

Alcoholic Liver Disease

Despite worldwide recognition of the role that alcohol plays in acute and chronic liver disease, alcoholic liver disease remains extraordinarily widespread. Alcohol is available worldwide, and most adults drink some amount of alcohol in a given year. It should be stressed that women tend to be more susceptible to the deleterious effects of alcohol than men.

Alcoholic liver disease exists on the spectrum. The first sign of liver disease in patients who consume alcohol is typically a so-called *fatty liver*. Fatty liver can develop after an episode of binge drinking or in the setting of chronic drinking. Microscopically, fatty liver appears as fat droplets within the cytosol of hepatocytes. Most patients with fatty liver from alcohol use are asymptomatic.

Fatty liver disease can progress to steatohepatitis, which implies inflammation as well as the presence of fat within the liver. Typically, a greater level of alcohol consumption is necessary to develop steatohepatitis. Patients with steatohepatitis are seen to have Mallory bodies on liver biopsy. A Mallory body, also known as *Mallory's hyaline*, is an intracellular inclusion body made up of keratin and other proteins. Patients with steatohepatitis are often seen to develop ballooning degeneration of hepatocytes, an inflammatory infiltrate, tissue necrosis, and fibrosis on liver biopsy. Many patients with steatohepatitis from alcohol use will have no symptoms, although some patients will develop right quadrant pain or other symptoms suggestive of liver disease. The classic laboratory abnormality in patients with steatohepatitis from alcohol is an aspartate aminotransferase (AST) and alanine aminotransferase (ALT) elevation where the ratio of AST to ALT is greater than 2:1.

If untreated, and if alcohol use continues, steatohepatitis can progress to alcoholic cirrhosis. Alcoholic cirrhosis has been and remains a common indication for liver transplantation.

The term *alcoholic hepatitis* is usually used to describe a specific syndrome seen in patients with alcoholic liver disease wherein patients develop a clinical picture consistent with acute hepatitis, often with hepatic decompensation. Patients with severe alcoholic hepatitis generally require hospitalization with intensive care unit and nutritional support. The management of severe alcoholic hepatitis has been, and remains, controversial. Although the use of corticosteroids in patients with severe alcoholic hepatitis has been studied in detail and appears to show benefit, a consultation with a dedicated hepatologist should be obtained before their initiation. Patients with jaundice, a prolonged prothrombin time, hepatic encephalopathy, or a high Model for End-Stage Liver Disease (MELD) score are at increased risk of dying from alcoholic hepatitis.

Nonalcoholic Fatty Liver Disease

Recent years have seen a great deepening in our understanding of the harm that fat can cause in the liver. *Nonalcoholic fatty liver disease* (NAFLD) is a general term that refers to the presence of fat in the liver and its sometimes harmful results. Nonalcoholic fatty liver refers to the presence of fat in the liver without attendant inflammation. Nonalcoholic steatohepatitis (NASH) refers to the accumulation of fat within the liver that is not felt to be due to alcohol use with resulting inflammation in the liver that, if chronic and untreated, can lead to cirrhosis. For many years, the degree of damage that fat could cause in the liver was unknown or, at best, poorly understood, and many physicians who saw patients with NASH and/or NASH-related cirrhosis often falsely suspected that patients were actually alcohol abusers.

Major risk factors for NAFLD include (but are not limited to) the following:

- Insulin resistance
- Factors associated with metabolic syndrome (ie, diabetes, obesity, hyperlipidemia, and hypertension)
- Elevated body mass index (bone mineral density)

- Chronically elevated serum aminotransferase levels
- Family history of diabetes, usually type 2
- High-fructose diet
- Choline deficiency

Diagnosis of Nonalcoholic Fatty Liver Disease/Nonalcoholic Steatohepatitis

Patients with suspected NAFLD/NASH often undergo noninvasive imaging such as abdominal ultrasound, CT scans, and/or MRI, all of which can disclose the presence of fat in the liver. A liver biopsy is sometimes performed to evaluate the severity of inflammation and fibrosis that are present. A special type of ultrasound called *elastography* can also give information about the presence of fibrosis in the liver without the need for a biopsy.

Treatments for NAFLD/NASH include the following:

- Weight loss (either through dieting or weight loss surgery)
- Increased exercise levels
- Dietary modification
- Insulin-sensitizing drugs
- Look for and treat any coexisting cardiovascular disease

These treatments may reduce fat in the liver, may reduce inflammation, and may reduce the risk of progressing to cirrhosis.

Autoimmune Hepatitis

Autoimmune hepatitis, as the name implies, stems from the patient's own immune system attacking their own liver, causing inflammation and hepatitis. The exact cause of autoimmune hepatitis remains unknown. The disease is more commonly seen in women than in men and is thought to arise through some sort of environmental trigger. Patients may have a predisposition to autoimmune diseases because many patients with auto-immune hepatitis also have a history of other autoimmune diseases.

Most patients with autoimmune hepatitis have the so-called *type 1* form of the disease. These patients have positive testing for autoimmune blood markers including antismooth muscle antibody and antinuclear antibody. Type 1 autoimmune hepatitis generally affects adults, whereas type 2 autoimmune hepatitis generally affects younger patients, typically children to teenagers. Patients with autoimmune hepatitis tend to have high circulating immunoglobulin levels.

The clinical presentation of autoimmune hepatitis can be variable. Some patients will present with signs of acute hepatitis including markedly elevated transaminase levels, jaundice, fatigue, etc. These patients tend to have disproportionately elevated AST and ALT levels, whereas their alkaline phosphatase level tends to be relatively low. Other patients can present in the setting of minimal symptoms with signs of advanced liver disease, including cirrhosis. Some of these patients may have been sick for months or years without becoming aware of an under-lying illness. Occasionally, patients with autoimmune hepatitis can present with an episode of gastrointestinal bleeding from portal hypertension.

Patients with autoimmune hepatitis are generally treated with immunosuppressants to good effect. Steroids and/or steroid-sparing agents such as azathioprine are commonly used, and a variety of treatment protocols exist. Most patients respond well, and treatment is typically of long duration.

Primary Biliary Cholangitis

Primary biliary cholangitis (formerly known as *primary biliary cirrhosis*), like autoimmune hepatitis, is a chronic liver disease that more typically affects women than men and is believed to have an autoimmune component. Patients with primary biliary cirrhosis classically lose their interlobular bile ducts due to chronic inflammation and develop jaundice and cirrhosis. Again, as is seen in autoimmune hepatitis, patients with primary biliary cholangitis often have a history of other autoimmune diseases. Patients typically have an elevated alkaline phosphatase that is disproportionately high. Other liver chemistries can be elevated as well. The classic blood test to check in patients with suspected primary biliary cirrhosis is an antimitochondrial antibody level. A positive antimitochondrial antibody test in a patient with clinical signs and symptoms of primary biliary cirrhosis is diagnostic for the disease.

Patients with primary biliary cholangitis often progress to chronic jaundice with accompanying pruritus. The pruritus of primary biliary cholangitis can be severe and debilitating. Other clinical features of primary biliary cholangitis include fatigue, fat-soluble vitamin deficiencies due to bile salt metabolism disruption, cutaneous cholesterol deposits known as *xanthelasmas* (often present under the eyes or on the extensor surfaces, such as the elbows and knees), and osteopenia or osteoporosis. Liver biopsy in patients with primary biliary cholangitis often reveals a lymphocytic infiltrate producing destruction of small bile ducts known as a *florid duct lesion*.

The mainstay of treatment for patients with primary biliary cholangitis is the drug ursodeoxycholic acid, generally dosed at 13 to 15 mg/kg/day. This agent has been shown to slow the progression of primary biliary cholangitis and can improve clinical and laboratory findings of cholestasis. Many patients with primary biliary cholangitis ultimately require liver transplantation.

Budd-Chiari Syndrome

Budd-Chiari syndrome is a vascular disease of the liver that warrants brief discussion. Budd-Chiari syndrome refers to hepatic venous outflow obstruction. This can occur within the hepatic veins themselves or within the inferior vena cava. Patients with Budd-Chiari syndrome can present acutely in the setting of a new hepatic venous outflow obstruction or after the obstruction itself has been long-standing. Many patients with Budd-Chiari syndrome have an underlying hypercoagulable state that leads to the formation of a clot within the hepatic venous system or an underlying disease that promotes clot formation, such as malignancy or severe infection. Patients may present with abdominal pain, ascites, gastrointestinal bleeding from a portal hypertensive source, hepatomegaly, and/or splenomegaly. If the thrombus is acute, patients may be candidates for thrombolytic agents, although this is rarely performed. Typically, patients with Budd-Chiari syndrome are managed via anticoagulation to prevent further clot formation and/or clot extension, TIPS placement to manage portal hypertension, and/or liver transplantation.

VIRAL HEPATITIS

Viral hepatitis is something that you need to understand if you will be seeing patients with gastrointestinal disease. Viral hepatitis is incredibly common and, unfortunately, somewhat complicated. Viral hepatitis can lead to both acute liver disease (up to and including fulminant hepatic failure requiring emergent liver transplantation), as well as chronic liver disease, cirrhosis, and HCC.

Do not be alarmed if this information seems somewhat complicated to you; even experienced physicians often need to check the reference books with regard to viral hepatitis from time to time. There is a lot of information to cover, and it is important to keep it all straight.

Hepatitis A Virus

Hepatitis A virus is a single-stranded RNA virus. Hepatitis A only leads to acute hepatitis. There is no chronic form of hepatitis A; you have either never had hepatitis A, have active hepatitis A, have had hepatitis A, or have been vaccinated for hepatitis A. You cannot acquire hepatitis A for a second time. Hepatitis A is usually transmitted orally through contaminated food or water supplies, but it can also be transmitted sexually.

In industrialized nations, hepatitis A is relatively rare. In developing nations, hepatitis A is extremely common, with a very high percentage of the population being exposed to the virus in childhood. In the United States and Europe, a vaccination for hepatitis A is widely available and leads to lasting immunity.

Clinically, patients typically get sick from hepatitis A several weeks after infection. Patients can develop malaise, flu-like symptoms, and jaundice. A small subset of patients who develop hepatitis A (usually less than 1%) will go on to develop fulminant hepatic failure and will need to be considered for emergency liver transplantation. Patients with fulminant hepatic failure from hepatitis A will typically die without liver transplantation.

There are 2 variant clinical pictures of hepatitis A that you should be familiar with. The first of these involves a long period of jaundice after hepatitis A infection. This is referred to as *prolonged cholestasis* (a fancy word for jaundice). During the recovery from hepatitis A infection, patients with prolonged cholestasis may experience months of jaundice even though they have otherwise resolved their hepatitis A infection. These patients may have an elevated alkaline phosphatase blood level as well. Treatment is usually supportive, and the jaundice will fade slowly over time (to the patient's relief!).

The second clinical variant of hepatitis A infection involves a clinical relapse of the disease weeks or months after the initial infection. Again, treatment is supportive unless patients develop fulminant hepatic failure.

Hepatitis B Virus

Hepatitis B virus is a major global health problem. Hundreds of millions of people around the world are infected with hepatitis B. In contrast to hepatitis A, hepatitis B virus can result in both acute and chronic infection. Chronic infection with hepatitis B is a major cause of cirrhosis and HCC worldwide as well as a major public health concern.

Hepatitis B virus is a double-stranded DNA virus. The virus comes in several forms, referred to as *genotypes*. Genotypes B, C, and D are typically seen in Asians; genotype A is most commonly seen in the United States among non-Asian patients.

Hepatitis B is typically spread through sexual contact and/or intravenous drug abuse. The virus is also commonly spread vertically via mother-to-child transmission, usually at the time of delivery. Hepatitis B can also be spread through contaminated blood products.

Clinically, patients with hepatitis B typically develop symptoms months after the initial infection. Malaise, flu-like symptoms, and right upper quadrant abdominal pain (often with associated jaundice) are commonly encountered, although some patients never develop jaundice during the acute infection. Fulminant hepatic failure can also develop from acute hepatitis B infection, but this is rare.

Patients with hepatitis B can either go on to clear the virus or develop chronic hepatitis B infection. The younger you are when you are exposed to hepatitis B virus, the more likely you are to develop chronic infection.

The blood test used to evaluate and monitor patients with hepatitis B exposure is somewhat complex. Once patients are infected with hepatitis B, they will have positive tests for the hepatitis B virus core protein antibody (HBcAb), hepatitis B virus e-antigen (HBeAg), and hepatitis B virus surface antigen (HBsAg). Patients will also develop positive testing for hepatitis B virus DNA. Patients who clear the virus develop positive testing for hepatitis B virus surface antibody (HBsAb). Once you develop HBsAb, you have cleared the infection and are cured. You cannot have a positive HBsAb test and still have active hepatitis B. In fact, the widely available vaccine for hepatitis B confers patients a positive HBsAb test as well.

Patients with chronic hepatitis B virus infection usually have positive testing for hepatitis B virus DNA, HBsAg, and the chronic form of the anti–hepatitis B virus core protein antibody (known as *IgG HBcAb*), and they may or may not express HBeAg.

A full discussion of the management of chronic hepatitis B is beyond this handbook, but you should know that there are both injectable and oral agents available for patients with chronic hepatitis B. The injectable agent interferon alfa and many oral antiviral agents are widely used around the world in an attempt to clear patients of hepatitis B virus and develop a positive HBsAb test. You should know that the virus is difficult to eradicate; many patients never clear the virus, and many patients require years of therapy to achieve a meaningful response.

Hepatitis C Virus

The hepatitis C virus is also an RNA virus. Like hepatitis B, hepatitis C is a major worldwide health problem. Infection with hepatitis C virus is a major cause of cirrhosis and HCC around the world. Hepatitis C infection is also a leading indication for liver transplantation in the United States.

Hepatitis C is transmitted via intravenous drug use, infected blood products, and sexual exposure. Vertical transmission is also possible but rare.

Most patients who acquire hepatitis C virus infection never know that they have become infected. Patients may develop a short flu-like illness or no symptoms at all. If patients are diagnosed with acute hepatitis C virus infection, early treatment has a good chance of leading to clearance of the virus. Unfortunately, we rarely identify patients with acute hepatitis C virus infection. Twenty percent to 40% of patients with hepatitis C virus will spontaneously clear the infection on their own. Patients who clear the virus develop an anti–hepatitis C virus antibody but will have normal liver function and no detectable hepatitis C virus in their blood.

The remainder of patients who develop hepatitis C virus will go on to develop chronic infection. Chronic infection can manifest as elevated serum liver tests, including AST and ALT. Some patients can have completely normal liver blood test despite active hepatitis C infection. The virus can lead to chronic inflammation and over a period of decades will often lead to cirrhosis. Many patients never know they have acquired hepatitis C infection until they develop signs or symptoms of cirrhosis. Other patients discover they have hepatitis C infection while attempting to donate blood (at which time the blood is screened) or when undergoing an insurance physical (during which time abnormal liver chemistries can be detected).

Treatment

The development of effective medications to treat hepatitis C can, without hyperbole, be considered one of the greatest triumphs of modern medicine. Treatments for hepatitis C were in their infancy 20 years ago, with high rates of side effects and low rates of cure (cure is also known as a *sustained viral response*).

Modern treatments for hepatitis C are easy to take and have extremely high rates of sustained viral response. A full description of the many different regimens to treat hepatitis C is beyond the scope of this book, but there are regimens that are specific for different genotypes of hepatitis C and regimens that are effective against all genotypes of hepatitis C. Most regimens involve 1 to 3 tablets a day, taken for 8 to 16 weeks, of 2 to 4 different medications dosed together. These regimens are sometimes modified for patients with cirrhosis. Most patients who undergo these treatments are effectively cured of their hepatitis C disease.

Hepatitis D Virus

Hepatitis D virus is yet another RNA virus. The most important thing to understand about the hepatitis D virus is that it can only make you ill if you are infected with the hepatitis B virus as well. The hepatitis D virus needs the hepatitis B virus to replicate; if you do not have infection with hepatitis B, you cannot become sick from the hepatitis D virus. Patients with acute infection from both hepatitis D and hepatitis B virus often develop severe acute hepatitis. Patients may have a fluctuating course with periods of improvement followed by significant worsening of their liver function and liver blood tests.

Patients with severe acute coinfection from both hepatitis D and hepatitis B virus infection are at high risk of developing fulminant hepatic failure and dying. In contrast, patients who already have chronic hepatitis B virus infection and who acquire hepatitis D virus may develop signs of acute hepatitis but are at lower risk of developing fulminant hepatic failure than patients who develop simultaneous infection with both viruses. Patients in this situation can develop chronic hepatitis B and D viral infection. There is no vaccine for hepatitis D virus.

Hepatitis E Virus

Hepatitis E virus is also an RNA virus (in case you had not noticed, the only DNA virus in this group is hepatitis B). Hepatitis E is common in Central America, the Middle East, and Asia, as well as parts of Africa. Hepatitis E virus infection is rare in the United States and Western Europe. Hepatitis E is generally spread through fecal-oral contact (yuck!). Patients can develop symptoms weeks or months after hepatitis E virus infection, again with flu-like or vague symptoms. Patients can develop jaundice and abnormal liver tests as well. Similar to hepatitis A virus infection, prolonged cholestasis can develop after infection with the hepatitis E virus. There is no chronic hepatitis E virus infection; patients either clear the virus and recover normal levels of liver function or go on to develop fulminant hepatic failure (which is rare). There is no vaccine for hepatitis E.

HEPATOCELLULAR CANCER

HCC is the term used to describe primary cancers of the liver. HCC is extremely common worldwide. Furthermore, patients with cirrhosis are at a markedly increased risk of developing HCC. All patients with cirrhosis, regardless of the etiology, are at increased risk of developing HCC when compared with the general population. As hepatitis C and hepatitis B infections have become alarmingly widespread around the world, the incidence of HCC has risen proportionately.

All patients with cirrhosis need to undergo periodic screening for HCC. The most cost-effective strategy involves right upper quadrant ultrasound examinations every 6 to 12 months in patients with established cirrhosis (Figure 5-2). Furthermore, the serum tumor marker known as *alpha-fetoprotein* should be followed in these

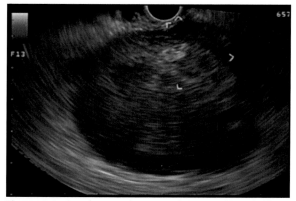

Figure 5-2. An ultrasound image of a 7-cm hepatocellular carcinoma.

patients as well. A rise in the alpha-fetoprotein level, especially in the context of a new lesion seen on ultrasound, is often diagnostic of HCC. Some centers use CT scanning as well as MRI scanning to screen patients for HCC.

It is worth mentioning briefly that not all patients with HCC have cirrhosis (although the majority of them do). Sometimes patients without any underlying liver disease can develop a sporadic HCC, and patients with viral hepatitis in the absence of cirrhosis can also develop HCC. For example, a patient with chronic hepatitis B without evidence of cirrhosis may develop HCC. In patients who do not have cirrhosis but who do develop HCC, primary resection of the tumor can often be performed. This is generally not true in patients with underlying cirrhosis; cirrhotic patients with HCC usually need to be evaluated for liver transplantation.

Not all patients with cirrhosis and HCC can undergo liver transplantation. Some patients develop multifocal tumors as well as large tumors (greater than 5 cm). Current practice dictates that patients with a single HCC

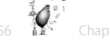
less than 5 cm in size or up to 3 HCCs less than 3 cm in size can be considered for liver transplantation. This rule is known as the *Milan criteria*.

Sometimes patients with cirrhosis have a tumor burden that exceeds the Milan criteria. Some of these patients can be made into surgical candidates for liver transplantation via undergoing one or more of several available treatments in an attempt to shrink their tumor size (or sizes) to allow them to fit under the umbrella of the Milan criteria. Interventional radiologists can attempt to treat these patients using techniques such as radiofrequency ablation and/or chemoembolization.

Patients with underlying cirrhosis who do go on to develop HCC may notice a rapid clinical decompensation without an obvious precipitating cause. Any rapid downturn in a patient with known cirrhosis should prompt consideration and investigation for the development of HCC.

LIVER TRANSPLANTATION

Liver transplantation, for lack of a more scientific description, is a big deal. Liver transplantation requires specialized hospitals with specialized surgeons, liver transplant hepatologists, intensive care units, pulmonologists, social workers, interventional gastroenterologists, interventional radiologists, and anesthesiologists, among others. The vast majority of hospitals in the United States cannot perform liver transplantation; rather, specialized centers around the country exist in order to coordinate the care of liver transplantation patients more centrally. If you are not practicing at a liver transplant center but you are taking care of patients with gastrointestinal disease in your hospital, you need to know where the nearest liver transplant center is and how to reach them for both routine and emergent cases.

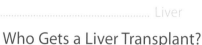

Who Gets a Liver Transplant?

Patients can undergo liver transplantation for a variety of clinical indications. The most common reason that patients undergo liver transplantation is cirrhosis with evidence of decompensated disease. Patients can also undergo transplantation for acute liver disease, again with signs of decompensation up to and including fulminant hepatic failure. Some reasons for acute liver transplantation would include liver failure from acetaminophen overdose, acute hepatitis A or B virus infection with fulminant hepatic failure, and severe alcoholic hepatitis.

In addition to severe underlying liver disease, patients being considered for liver transplantation have to have a solid social support network (to help deal with the medical burdens of liver transplantation), the financial ability to help pay for the cost of the transplant itself as well as aftercare including immunosuppressive medications, and a lack of significant contraindications to liver transplantation (eg, active drug use, active alcohol use).

Patients with underlying alcoholic cirrhosis generally have to be able to prove sobriety for at least 6 months before being considered for liver transplantation. Some centers use random alcohol and drug testing in patients with a known history of alcohol and/or substance abuse. Patients with acute alcoholic hepatitis with evidence of decompensation can undergo liver transplantation without a 6-month period of sobriety as a lifesaving measure.

Model for End-Stage Liver Disease Scores

MELD scores are used in most centers as a tool to gauge the severity of a patient's underlying liver disease. MELD scores can be applied to patients with acute or chronic liver disease. The MELD score uses certain easily obtained parameters to assess the patient's overall degree

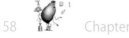
of liver function and health. The MELD score is calculated as follows (Of note, there is a correction factor for patients who have to undergo dialysis):

$$MELD = 3.78(Ln \ serum \ bilirubin \ [mg/dL]) + 11.2(Ln \ INR) + 9.57(Ln \ serum \ creatinine \ [mg/dL]) + 6.43.$$

The MELD score formula is not something you have to memorize; you can go to many websites that will calculate the MELD score for you such as http://www.mayoclinic.org/meld/mayomodel6.html. The MELD score has largely replaced the previously used Child-Turcotte-Pugh score to measure the severity of underlying liver disease. The higher the MELD score, the higher the risk of dying while waiting for liver transplantation. The MELD score has become popular as an objective means of assessing the severity of the illness while placing patients on the liver transplantation waiting list.

Surgical Options for Patients Undergoing Liver Transplantation

Patients undergoing liver transplantation can do so via a variety of techniques. It should be noted that all liver transplantation is referred to as *orthotopic*. Orthotopic refers to the fact that the old liver must be removed, and the new liver must be placed in the same location as the old liver in order to function. Although this is true for liver transplantation, it is not true for all surgical transplantations. Kidney and pancreas transplantations often involve placement of the new transplanted organ into the patient's pelvis (and not at the site of the native kidney or pancreas). These types of transplants are referred to as *heterotopic transplantations*.

Most patients who undergo liver transplantation have their liver removed and receive an entire liver from another person. Obviously, in such situations, the donor of the liver must no longer be alive. Most donor livers come from trauma victims, from people who have committed suicide by methods such as drug overdose (by agents not harmful to the liver), or from patients who are declared legally brain dead.

Another option involves removal of the entire diseased liver and the transplant of part of a liver (usually the left lobe) from a living person. A person who donates the left lobe will usually regenerate a full-size liver over time. The transplanted left lobe is often adequate to provide full liver function for the transplant recipient. Sometimes neonates or children who need to undergo liver transplantation can receive a portion of a liver from a parent or a sibling. This is referred to as *living-donor liver transplantation*. This type of transplantation is not without risk to the donor, and potential donors must undergo a rigorous screening process to ensure that they are fully aware of the risks involved.

Life After Liver Transplantation

Most patients who successfully undergo liver transplantation experience a dramatic improvement in their quality of life. For some of these patients, liver transplantation means an end to all liver disease. Patients with hereditary hemochromatosis, Wilson's disease, and alpha-1 antitrypsin deficiency, for example, become free of not only their diseased liver but also their underlying disease process. These diseases do not recur after liver transplantation. Other diseases such as chronic hepatitis B and C infection, primary sclerosing cholangitis, and autoimmune hepatitis can recur after transplantation. Some patients can live long enough to develop cirrhosis in a new liver and undergo a second transplantation down the road.

Patients who do undergo liver transplantation usually need to take immunosuppressive medications for life. Many patients who undergo liver transplantation can experience rejection of the new liver, and rejection can be acute or chronic. Patients can develop bile duct strictures and/or leaks that may require endoscopic treatment, and patients can develop postoperative vascular complications such as hepatic artery thrombosis, hepatic vein thrombosis, and hemorrhage. All of these problems can be managed, but some are more severe and can result in failure of the transplanted liver itself and require retransplantation.

BIBLIOGRAPHY

Bari K, Garcia-Tsao G. Treatment of portal hypertension. *World J Gastroenterol.* 2012;18(11):1166-1175.

Bonder A, Afdhal N. Evaluation of liver lesions. *Clin Liver Dis.* 2012;16(2):271-283.

Kamath PS, Kim WR; Advanced Liver Disease Study Group. The model for end-stage liver disease (MELD). *Hepatology.* 2007;45(3):797-805.

Maggs JR, Suddle AR, Aluvihare V, Heneghan MA. Systematic review: the role of liver transplantation in the management of hepatocellular carcinoma. *Aliment Pharmacol Ther.* 2012;35(10):1113-1134.

Singh T, Allende DS, McCullough AJ. Assessing liver fibrosis without biopsy in patients with HCV or NAFLD. *Cleve Clin J Med.* 2019;86(3):179-186.

Chapter 6

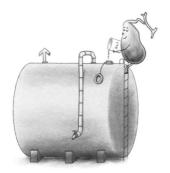

Gallbladder and Bile Ducts

It may seem odd to have this particular chapter (on the gallbladder and the bile ducts) and a separate chapter on the liver; aren't the gallbladder and the bile ducts really part of the liver? The answer is yes and no; the bile ducts are integrally related to the liver, and the gallbladder is functionally part of the biliary tree, but diseases of the gallbladder and the bile ducts are often thought about and treated separately from most other liver diseases. Of course, there is some overlap between the 2, and this chapter will reference some material we have already touched on in Chapter 5.

Adler DG. *The Little GI Book: An Easily Digestible Guide to Understanding Gastroenterology, Second Edition* (pp 161-191).
© 2020 Taylor & Francis Group.

ANATOMY

As discussed earlier, bile serves many functions, including aiding in fat digestion as well as removal of certain toxins from the body. Bile is manufactured in hepatocytes where it is transported into the smallest bile ducts—the bile canaliculi. These microscopic ducts drain into the small intrahepatic bile ducts. The intrahepatic bile ducts on the right side of the liver eventually coalesce into the right hepatic duct. The intrahepatic bile ducts on the left side of the liver eventually coalesce into the left hepatic duct. The left and right hepatic ducts join in a region known as the *hilum* to form the common hepatic duct. The common hepatic duct drains into the common bile duct (CBD), and the CBD drains into the duodenum through the sphincter of Oddi, which is contained within the major duodenal papilla (sometimes referred to as the *major papilla*, the *ampulla of Vater*, or simply as the *ampulla*; Figure 6-1).

The gallbladder serves as a reservoir for bile; bile is made by the liver 24 hours a day, but bile is primarily needed only after ingesting a meal. Thus, it makes sense to have a place to store bile so that when you eat a meal (especially a meal containing fatty foods), you have lots of bile ready to be secreted into the duodenum to mix with the food. Bile flows in and out of the gallbladder via the cystic duct. The cystic duct can join the CBD at a variety of locations, but in general the cystic duct joins the mid- to distal CBD. The act of eating a meal, especially a fatty meal, triggers the release of the hormones secretin and cholecystokinin. These hormones stimulate the gallbladder to contract and release bile into the duodenum via the biliary tree.

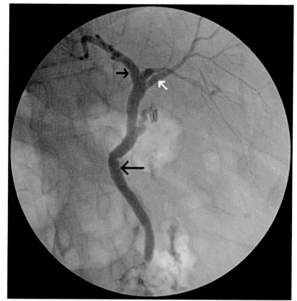

Figure 6-1. Normal bile ducts seen via endoscopic retrograde cholangiopancreatography (ERCP). The left and right hepatic ducts (small black arrow and small white arrow, respectively) drain into the common hepatic duct. The common hepatic ducts become the CBD (large black arrow), which drains into the duodenum at the bottom of the image. Note the clips across the cystic duct remnant, indicating prior cholecystectomy.

A FEW BRIEF WORDS ABOUT BILE METABOLISM

Bile consists of many different substances mixed together. Bile is predominantly made of water but also consists of bile acids (which, when joined to a positively charged ion, are known as *bile salts*), cholesterol, fat, mucus, and a few other trace ingredients. Bile salts are important in the breakdown in digestion of fats in the diet. Cholesterol is required for normal health and function of cells, especially normal and healthy cell walls. Bilirubin, the principal breakdown product of heme in red blood cells, is also excreted in bile. Bile is also a means for certain drugs and other chemicals to be excreted into the bowel so that they can be removed from the body via feces. The process by which these elements are made water soluble for secretion into bile and thus out of the body is known as *glucuronidation*.

Of note, the bile acid pool is constantly recycled through the liver and small bowel via a process known as *enterohepatic circulation*. Bile acids synthesized in the liver are secreted into the small bowel through the bile ducts. Some of these bile salts are lost in stool, whereas others are reabsorbed in the ileum and transported back to the liver via the portal venous system for further use and circulation. Diseases that damage the ileum, classically Crohn's disease, can produce a net loss of bile salts with disordered enterohepatic circulation and are often associated with a form of diarrhea known as *bile acid diarrhea*. Bile acid diarrhea can be treated with bile salt sequestrants, such as the drug cholestyramine.

SOME CONFUSING TERMINOLOGY TO UNDERSTAND

When discussing diseases of the gallbladder and the bile ducts, one quickly encounters some tricky terminology. In truth, these terms make perfect sense from a technical point of view, but they take some getting used to. The following are some common terms that you will encounter when dealing with diseases of the bile duct and their treatments:

- **Cholelithiasis:** Gallbladder stones (chole = bile, lith = stone)
- **Choledocholithiasis:** Bile duct stones (chole = bile, docho = duct, lith = stone); get it?
- **Cholecystitis:** An inflamed gallbladder, usually implying infection as well
- **Cholangitis:** Inflammation of the bile ducts, usually implying infection as well
- **Cholecystectomy:** Surgical removal of the gallbladder
- **Cholangiography:** A picture of the bile ducts (obtained via ERCP, magnetic resonance cholangiopancreatography [MRCP], etc)
- **Cholangioscopy:** A means of viewing the inside of the bile ducts via the use of microscopic cameras
- **Choledochoduodenostomy:** A hole, naturally occurring or surgically created, between the bile ducts and the duodenum
- **Choledochojejunostomy:** A hole, almost always surgically created, between the bile ducts and the jejunum
- **Hepaticojejunostomy:** A surgical communication between the bile ducts (usually at the level of the hilum or common hepatic duct) and the jejunum; this is similar to a choledochojejunostomy but often involves removal of the CBD as well (as is performed in a pancreaticoduodenectomy [Whipple procedure] for pancreatic cancer)
- **Choledochocele:** A cyst of the bile ducts, often premalignant in nature
- **Cholangiocarcinoma:** Cancer of the bile ducts
- **Gallbladder cancer:** Gallbladder cancer (I thought we could finish with an easy one!)

GALLSTONES AND
GALLSTONE DISEASE

Gallstones and gallstone disease remain incredibly common. A very high percentage of the population will have stones in their gallbladder at any given time. Because so many people have stones in their gallbladder, even if only a small percentage of those stones become symptomatic or clinically relevant, it translates to a large number of patients needing clinical care for gallstones and gallstone-related diseases.

Gallstones can be of several varieties; most are made of cholesterol or cholesterol mixed with other substances, including bile salts and biliary pigments. Some stones that are just made of pigment are encountered as well. Patients usually develop gallstones in the setting of some abnormality of biliary function and/or metabolism. The most common cause of gallstones is supersaturation of bile with cholesterol. Cholesterol can become concentrated in bile during pregnancy, as a consequence of genetics or diet, or for idiopathic reasons. Supersaturated bile can precipitate out of solution and form cholesterol crystals that can ultimately become stones. Other key factors that can lead to the formation of gallstones include poor gallbladder contractility (known as *gallbladder hypomotility*) that leads to stasis of bile in the gallbladder and the presence of bacteria within bile. Some patients have many risk factors for gallstones (family history, pregnancy, and documented gallbladder hypomotility on special testing), whereas other patients with stones will have no identifiable risk factors. Many patients with gallstones will live their whole lives and never develop any symptoms; this is referred to as *asymptomatic cholelithiasis* and generally requires no treatment. When stones cause symptoms, intervention is usually warranted.

BILIARY COLIC

The term *biliary colic* refers to the typical pain encountered in patients with cholelithiasis in the absence of cholecystitis. Biliary colic often manifests as intense right upper quadrant abdominal pain that can last for hours at a time. The pain may be triggered by eating a fatty meal or certain trigger foods that may not be fatty at all. The pain may radiate to the back or the shoulder or may not radiate at all. Patients with biliary colic typically have multiple attacks and may develop a fear of eating certain foods that they think may trigger an attack. The pain of biliary colic usually resolves spontaneously. From a pathophysiology point of view, the exact cause of biliary colic is not always clear. In some patients, it is thought that biliary colic is due to a stone obstructing the neck of the gallbladder combined with the gallbladder attempting to contract against a functional obstruction. Other patients can have symptomatic biliary colic without clear evidence of an obstructing stone in the gallbladder. Biliary colic may also be secondary to a gallstone transiting the cystic duct en route to the CBD. Some patients may have cystic duct stones that never fully reach the CBD that may cause intermittent obstruction of the cystic duct itself.

CHOLECYSTITIS

As defined previously, cholecystitis implies inflammation of the gallbladder. Cholecystitis also often typically implies infection of the gallbladder. Calculous cholecystitis implies infection of the gallbladder with concomitant stone disease, whereas acalculous cholecystitis implies infection in the absence of stone disease.

Patients with cholecystitis often complain of intense right upper quadrant pain, fever, and worsening of their pain when taking a deep breath (due to pressure on the gallbladder and liver during the expansion of the lungs during inhalation) known as *Murphy's sign*. Patients with cholecystitis may also have epigastric pain that radiates to their back, which may be from the cholecystitis itself or due to concomitant pancreatitis caused by choledocholithiasis. It is important to emphasize that patients with acute cholecystitis present along a spectrum; some patients with acute cholecystitis will only appear mildly ill, whereas others will have an acute life-threatening process with signs of systemic infection/sepsis, shock, hypotension, etc.

Patients with cholecystitis may or may not be jaundiced. In some cases, jaundice can occur in the absence of biliary obstruction. In these patients, the jaundice is likely secondary due to acute infection. On the other hand, some patients with cholecystitis will have simultaneous choledocholithiasis with acute biliary obstruction. These patients really have 2 problems that need addressing: the gallbladder itself, which likely needs to be removed, and the CBD stones, which almost always need to be removed.

From the laboratory point of view, patients with cholecystitis will typically have an elevated white blood cell count and abnormal liver chemistries. Patients may have a disproportionately elevated alkaline phosphatase level, and elevated transaminases are commonly seen in the setting. As mentioned earlier, it is always important to check for concomitant pancreatitis by checking serum amylase and lipase levels.

From an imaging point of view, the best first test to order is right upper quadrant ultrasound. Right upper quadrant ultrasound examination can tell you whether or not the gallbladder looks normal or inflamed. Cholecystitis can manifest on right quadrant ultrasound as a gallbladder with surrounding fluid (pericholecystic fluid), gallbladder wall thickening, or air in the gallbladder (which could imply gas-forming organisms within the gallbladder or gallbladder perforation). A right upper quadrant ultrasound will also almost always be able to detect cholelithiasis. Beyond the gallbladder itself, a right upper quadrant ultrasound will often be able to identify the CBD and measure its diameter. Bile duct dilation in the setting of cholecystitis is suggestive, but not conclusive, for choledocholithiasis. Occasionally, right upper quadrant ultrasound can directly visualize choledocholithiasis, but this is the exception and not the rule.

Most patients with acute cholecystitis are treated surgically via cholecystectomy. In the modern era, most patients undergo laparoscopic cholecystectomy; so-called *open cholecystectomy* is typically reserved for patients with challenging anatomy or those in whom laparoscopic approaches are unsuccessful. During the cholecystectomy, the surgeon may perform an intra-operative cholangiogram. This involves placing a small catheter into the cystic duct and injecting contrast dye into the biliary tree to obtain an image of the biliary tree. If the bile duct is seen to be clear and free of stones, no further biliary intervention is generally required. If the intraoperative cholangiogram demonstrates what appear to be CBD stones, these can either be removed directly by the surgeon during the cholecystectomy (which is rarely performed for technical reasons) or at a later time via ERCP (which we do all the time).

Sometimes patients with acute cholecystitis are simply too sick to undergo cholecystectomy via surgery. This can occur if patients have other comorbidities and/or conditions that would make surgery too risky (eg, a very recent acute heart attack or stroke). These patients are generally treated with systemic antibiotics and some form of gallbladder drainage. Gallbladder drainage in patients too sick to undergo surgery for acute cholecystitis can be performed by percutaneous or endoscopic means. A percutaneous catheter can be placed into the gallbladder by an interventional radiologist. This is known as a *cholecystostomy tube*. Cholecystostomy tubes work well and can help treat the infection in the gallbladder by providing drainage. However, cholecystostomy tubes are very unpopular with patients because they are often permanent; are uncomfortable; and can interfere with activities such as bathing, intimacy, and even dressing and showering.

Endoscopic approaches to drain the gallbladder exist as well. One approach is to access the gallbladder during ERCP and place a stent into the gallbladder to drain it. In this procedure, a guidewire is threaded through the cystic duct and into the gallbladder via a catheter placed into the bile duct. A thin plastic stent is then advanced over this wire so that the gallbladder drains through this stent down to the duodenum. This provides internal drainage and spares the patient a percutaneous cholecystostomy tube.

Another endoscopic approach to treating patients with cholecystitis who are not surgical candidates (which is also discussed in Chapter 8) is a transluminal gallbladder drainage procedure. As the name implies, this involves direct drainage of the gallbladder via a puncture of the stomach or small bowel that connects the luminal gastrointestinal tract to the gallbladder directly. Special stents are used to keep the gallbladder connected to the stomach or small bowel, usually forever. These patients also achieve internal drainage and can skip having a percutaneous cholecystostomy tube placed.

CHOLEDOCHOLITHIASIS

Choledocholithiasis refers to CBD stones (Figure 6-2). Most patients with CBD stones become symptomatic at some point and require treatment. CBD stones can

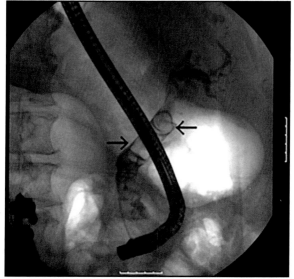

Figure 6-2. Stones seen as "filling defects" (arrows) via ERCP.

produce symptoms identical to biliary colic from chole-lithiasis. Patients may also develop jaundice and/or acute pancreatitis. Untreated chronic obstruction from bile duct stones can lead to a chronic inflammatory condition of the bile ducts known as *secondary sclerosing cholangitis* (SSC).

CBD stones can often be suspected based on the patient's history, physical examination, and laboratory values. Patients will often have right upper quadrant pain, jaundice, and elevated alkaline phosphatase and liver chemistries. CBD stones can be directly visualized via a number of methods. Intraoperative cholangiogram, right upper quadrant ultrasound, magnetic resonance imaging with MRCP, ERCP, endoscopic ultrasound, and computed tomography scans can all definitively see CBD stones. Magnetic resonance imaging with MRCP

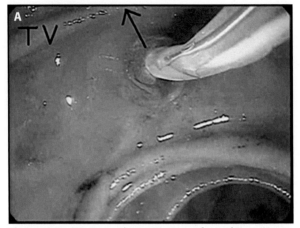

Figure 6-3. (A) An endoscopic view of a sphincterotome in the major papilla in a patient about to undergo biliary sphincterotomy. The arrow shows the direction of the cut. The transverse fold (TV) is often used as a marker in deciding how large a sphincterotomy to create. (*continued*)

and endoscopic ultrasound are the best noninvasive and minimally invasive technologies, respectively, for looking for bile duct stones, and these can be considered comparable diagnostic tests.

CBD stones are typically removed via ERCP. As discussed in Chapter 8, ERCP allows physicians to access the bile ducts endoscopically. In almost all cases, a biliary sphincterotomy must be performed before removing CBD stones via ERCP. This creates a much more generous communication between the distal CBD and the duodenum for stone extraction (Figure 6-3).

Most bile duct stones can be easily removed via ERCP (Figure 6-4). In approximately 90% of patients, all stones can be removed in one procedure. Patients with many stones, large stones, impacted stones, or intrahepatic

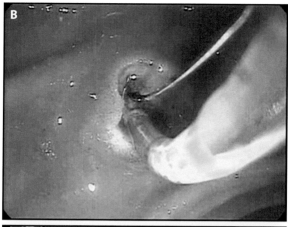

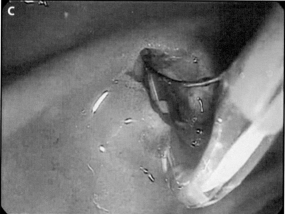

Figure 6-3 (continued). (B) Using electrocautery, the sphincterotomy is created. (C) Final appearance of the completed sphincterotomy.

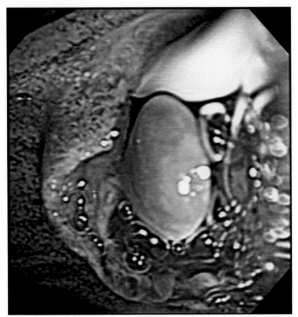

Figure 6-4. A stone in the duodenum after extraction from the bile duct during ERCP. Note the fresh sphincterotomy around the stone.

stones may need multiple procedures or more aggressive techniques to achieve stone clearance. Rarely, stones cannot be removed via ERCP for technical reasons and must be removed via surgery.

BILE LEAKS

Bile leaks occur when there has been some disruption in the biliary tree. Bile leaks allow bile to spill into the abdomen where it collects and causes pain and

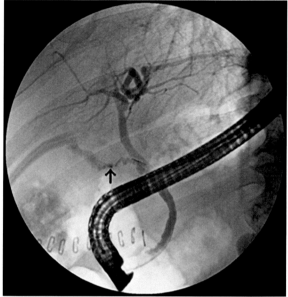

Figure 6-5. A cholangiogram obtained via ERCP showing a bile leak from the cystic duct remnant after cholecystectomy. Note the contrast dye freely flowing out of the biliary tree into the abdomen (arrow).

inflammation, collectively referred to as *bile peritonitis*. A collection of free bile within the abdomen is known as a *biloma* and can become infected. Bile leaks commonly occur after surgical intervention on the bile ducts, most commonly after cholecystectomy, although they can occur after liver resections, liver transplant, etc. In a typical postcholecystectomy bile leak, the cystic duct remnant is inadequately closed via sutures or clips placed during surgery. This creates a free opening between the biliary tree and the abdomen (Figure 6-5). Liquid bile will flow down the biliary tree and exit the bile duct via the pathway of least resistance. In a normal patient, the pathway of least resistance is down through the biliary tree toward the CBD and through the sphincter of Oddi into the duodenum. In a patient with a cystic duct leak, the path of least resistance is out through the cystic duct remnant (into the abdomen) and not the sphincter of Oddi.

The treatment of bile leaks is somewhat counterintuitive; one would imagine we would simply find the site of the leak and close it with a suture or a staple or some other mechanical device. Although this can be done, it is rarely performed in practice. Direct identification of the leak site with primary closure would require surgery, which most patients are eager to avoid if possible. Almost all bile leaks are managed endoscopically via ERCP. Patients with bile leaks typically undergo transampullary stent placement and/or biliary sphincterotomy. These approaches create a generous communication and promote flow between the biliary tree and the duodenum. This also makes the pathway of least resistance for bile flow to be to the duodenum and not out through the leak site. Once the flow of bile is diverted toward its normal route again, the leak site itself will slowly heal and close off over a period of several weeks. Treatment of bile leaks via a biliary stent placement alone, biliary sphincterotomy, or biliary stent placement combined with sphincterotomy are all viable options, and the decision of how to manage each leak is left to the individual endoscopist at the time of the ERCP. Also, most bile leaks can be treated electively and do not require emergent intervention. It is often more important to place a drain in the patient's abdomen to remove any bile that has accumulated there because the bile in the abdomen is really what makes patients feel very sick. These abdominal drains are usually placed by surgeons or interventional radiologists.

BILE DUCT STRICTURES

Bile duct strictures are a big problem and one that we encounter on a daily basis. Strictures of the bile duct often lead to clinical jaundice and symptoms of biliary obstruction (pruritus and so on) and warrant investigation. Bile duct strictures can be intrinsic or extrinsic in nature; intrinsic strictures arise from primary diseases of the bile ducts themselves, whereas extrinsic strictures are usually due to compression from another object or organ.

The 2 main tools used to treat biliary strictures are dilation and stenting, both of which are usually performed via endoscopy. Biliary strictures can be dilated using pneumatic or catheter-based dilators during ERCP. Biliary stricture dilation can also be performed during percutaneous biliary procedures performed by interventional radiologists. Stents can be temporary or permanent depending on the nature of the stricture and the patient's overall history (ie, a patient with an inflammatory stricture due to recent bile duct stone passage will likely be treated with a temporary plastic biliary stent, whereas a patient with metastatic pancreatic cancer and jaundice will usually be treated with a permanent self-expanding metal stent). If a stricture is malignant, usually dilation will not help in a lasting manner, and the patient just needs to be stented.

Bile duct strictures can arise from the following specific causes:

- **Pancreatic cancer:** The distal CBD runs through the head of the pancreas. Many pancreatic tumors occur in the head of the gland. As these tumors grow, they can extrinsically compress the distal CBD and lead to clinical jaundice and obstruction. When detected on imaging studies, simultaneous obstruction of the bile duct and the main pancreatic duct from a pancreatic head tumor is known as the *double-duct sign* (Figure 6-6).

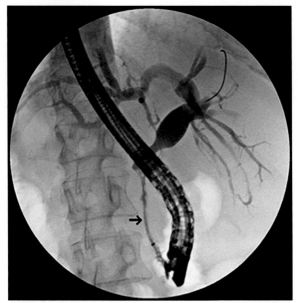

Figure 6-6. A malignant CBD stricture seen via ERCP in a patient with pancreatic cancer. The distal common duct is tightly stenosed (arrow), and the proximal intra- and extrahepatic ducts are all dilated.

- **Cholangiocarcinoma:** Primary bile duct cancer is referred to as *cholangiocarcinoma*. Cholangiocarcinoma usually results in an intrinsic biliary stricture. The most common location for bile duct stricture in patients with cholangiocarcinoma is at the common hepatic duct where it bifurcates into the left and right hepatic ducts (although cholangiocarcinoma can develop anywhere in the biliary tree). Patients can develop combined left- and right-sided biliary obstruction from a cholangiocarcinoma. Patients with combined left- and right-sided biliary obstruction from cholangiocarcinoma can be difficult to treat; it can sometimes be difficult to provide adequate biliary drainage to relieve their jaundice.

- **Primary sclerosing cholangitis (PSC):** PSC is a chronic inflammatory condition of the bile duct with associated liver dysfunction that often progresses to cirrhosis. Bile duct strictures in PSC are very common. More on this is covered later in this chapter.

- **Gallbladder cancer:** Primary tumors of the gallbladder, although rarely encountered, can obstruct the bile duct either by extrinsic compression or direct invasion.

- **Biliary surgery/surgical injury:** Many biliary strictures are postsurgical in nature. The blood flow to the bile ducts themselves is somewhat tenuous, and the bile ducts tolerate injury poorly. Thus, surgical injury to the bile ducts often results in the stricture. Common causes of biliary surgical injury include mechanical injury to the CBD or common hepatic duct during cholecystectomy (when the surgeon accidentally places a clip across the bile duct, accidentally cauterizes the bile duct, etc) or during liver transplantation. Most patients who undergo liver transplantation undergo the creation of what is known as a *primary duct-to-duct anastomosis*. This means that the CBD from the donor liver is sewn directly onto the recipient's native CBD with the 2 ducts forming a single pipe to carry bile from the liver to the duodenum. This anastomotic site is a common location for postsurgical strictures. Most anastomotic biliary strictures due to liver transplantation are treated with a combination of dilation and stenting and respond well to therapy. In contrast, injuries of the CBD that occur during cholecystectomy may be much more difficult to treat. Many of these postcholecystectomy injuries require multiple rounds of dilation and stenting, whereas others can only be repaired surgically (with a biliary bypass).

- **Bile duct inflammation:** Bile duct inflammation can lead to strictures anywhere in the biliary tree. The bile duct can become inflamed from a variety of causes, including choledocholithiasis, PSC or SSC, autoimmune cholangiography, and other causes. These can all lead to inflammatory strictures. Sometimes it can be difficult to distinguish an inflammatory stricture from a malignant stricture, and tissue sampling may be required to exclude malignancy.

- **Acute pancreatitis:** Inflammation of the pancreas can lead to extrinsic compression of the CBD as it courses through the pancreatic head. Many patients with acute pancreatitis will develop some degree of cholestasis even in the absence of choledocholithiasis. As the pancreatitis subsides and the swelling around the CBD resolves, the stricture generally disappears spontaneously. Sometimes patients with acute pancreatitis will develop pseudocysts that can cause long-lasting compression of the CBD and concomitant jaundice. In these cases, patients often receive biliary stents to relieve their jaundice. The pseudocysts may spontaneously resolve or require endoscopic and/or surgical drainage.

- **Chronic pancreatitis:** Patients with chronic pancreatitis may also develop CBD strictures due to extrinsic compression from inflammation and/or scarring and fibrosis of the pancreatic head.

Biliary strictures that arise in the setting of chronic pancreatitis may be extremely difficult to treat. Fibrosis in the pancreatic head due to chronic pancreatitis may be long-standing and may never resolve. Patients with biliary strictures from chronic pancreatitis often require one or more plastic biliary stents (placed side by side) in an attempt to provide both biliary drainage and biliary stricture dilation simultaneously. Some physicians use a covered self-expanding metal stent in an off-label manner in these patients to provide more long-lasting drainage and stricture dilation. Patients with calcific chronic pancreatitis who develop a biliary stricture are more likely to have a poor outcome. These patients may never resolve their stricture regardless of prolonged biliary stenting. Some patients with intractable biliary strictures from chronic pancreatitis have to undergo surgery (usually in the form of a biliary bypass) to definitively treat their biliary obstruction.

- **Metastatic cancer:** Patients with tumors that are metastatic to the liver (or, rarely, the pancreatic head) can develop a biliary stricture due to extrinsic compression from metastases. Patients in this situation are generally treated with biliary stents with good outcome.

- **Adenopathy:** Some patients will develop a biliary stricture due to extrinsic compression from a periductal lymph node. This can be seen in patients with advanced cancer and/or primary hematologic malignancies, such as lymphoma. These patients are typically treated with biliary stents. The stents can often be removed if the underlying adenopathy can be resolved via chemotherapy, radiation therapy, etc.

Primary Sclerosing Cholangitis

PSC is a chronic inflammatory condition of the bile ducts that often progresses to cirrhosis of the entire liver. PSC deserves special mention and more lengthy discussion than other bile duct diseases in this chapter given how many biliary complications can arise from PSC.

PSC has no known cause. It is strongly associated with inflammatory bowel disease, although a significant number of patients with PSC do not have any inflammatory bowel disease. PSC is more strongly associated with ulcerative colitis than Crohn's disease and more strongly associated with colitis than with small bowel disease in patients with inflammatory bowel disease. Most patients with inflammatory bowel disease never develop PSC, yet most patients with PSC have inflammatory bowel disease.

PSC leads to chronic inflammation of the intra- and extrahepatic biliary tree. There is a wide range of presentations in patients with PSC. Patients with PSC may have mild liver disease with normal liver chemistries or may have severe liver disease combining features of both biliary disease and cirrhosis with portal hypertension and profoundly abnormal liver chemistries. PSC remains a frequent indication for liver transplantation. PSC can recur after liver transplantation in the new donor liver.

Unfortunately, there is no medical therapy for patients with PSC. Many medications have been tried in patients with PSC, but none have been universally shown to significantly affect survival or improve the underlying liver and biliary disease. The only therapies that we have at the present time for patients with PSC include antibiotics to treat biliary infections, biliary interventions such as ERCP (to treat strictures, remove stones, etc), and surgery (partial hepatectomy to remove cancers of the bile ducts and/or liver transplantation).

Patients with PSC can develop a variety of complications, including the following:

- **Cholangitis:** This refers to a bacterial infection in the bile duct, usually due to a stricture blocking off one or more segments of the liver. This is treated via the use of antibiotics and a procedure to open up the duct stricture and drain it (usually via ERCP).

- **Bile duct strictures:** Bile duct strictures are a mainstay of disease in patients with PSC. Strictures can occur in the extra- and/or intrahepatic ducts, and patients with PSC often develop multiple strictures in the biliary tree simultaneously. A hallmark of patients with PSC is the development of the innumerable small intrahepatic ductal strictures (Figure 6-7). Patients may or may not develop jaundice from their strictures, but strictures that do result in jaundice are typically treated by biliary dilation, biliary stenting, or both. Sometimes patients with PSC will develop a very striking stricture known as a *dominant stricture*. The term *dominant stricture* is imprecise and to some extent unscientific but generally refers to a biliary stricture in a patient with PSC that appears concerning for malignancy (cholangiocarcinoma).

- **Cholangiocarcinoma:** Patients with PSC are at high risk for the development of cholangiocarcinoma. Patients with PSC are often surveyed by imaging and/or ERCP studies to evaluate them for concerning strictures or liver lesions that could represent cholangiocarcinoma. During these ERCP procedures, concerning biliary strictures can be brushed to collect cells, and the specimens can be sent for cytologic analysis to look for cancer. A relatively new but highly effective additional test that can be performed on cells obtained from biliary brushings in patients with PSC is known

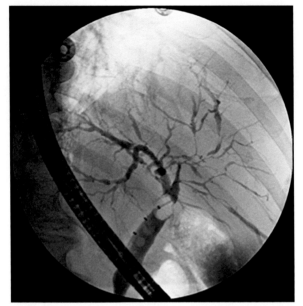

Figure 6-7. A cholangiogram obtained via ERCP in a patient with PSC. Note the innumerable intrahepatic duct strictures.

as *fluorescent in situ hybridization* (FISH). FISH testing specifically looks for aneuploidy within the cells obtained during the biliary brushing. The term *aneuploidy* refers to abnormal numbers of chromosomes within the cell (ie, each cell should have exactly 2 copies of each chromosome, no more and no less). Patients who have PSC with aneuploidy seen on biliary brushing via FISH are at high risk for harboring a cholangiocarcinoma.

- **Choledocholithiasis:** Patients with PSC often develop choledocholithiasis at some point in their disease. These bile duct stones are typically removed via ERCP.

- **Cirrhosis:** Most patients with PSC will eventually develop cirrhosis. In addition to the biliary complications of PSC, all of the typical complications of cirrhosis can also develop (eg, ascites, portal hypertension, varices).

PRIMARY SCLEROSING CHOLANGITIS LOOK-ALIKES

Several diseases can mimic PSC. These diseases can produce biliary ductal changes that can closely resemble PSC on a cholangiogram and on testing of liver chemistries.

- **SSC:** SSC refers to chronic biliary inflammation with an identifiable cause (in contrast to PSC, which is idiopathic). Most patients develop SSC due to untreated chronic obstruction of the bile duct. SSC can arise due to chronic choledocholithiasis or in patients who have biliary strictures that go untreated for a long period of time. SSC can develop in patients with postsurgical biliary strictures (ie, bile duct strictures that develop as a consequence of an injury that occurred during cholecystectomy), often unbeknownst to the patient. Sometimes patients have a temporary stent placed in their duct and fail to return to have it removed; a chronic indwelling stent like this can also lead to SSC over time.

- **HIV cholangiopathy:** As the name would imply, HIV cholangiopathy is a chronic inflammatory disease of the bile ducts seen in patients with HIV/AIDS. HIV cholangiopathy can closely mimic PSC in terms of its appearance during ERCP. Unlike PSC, HIV cholangiopathy often leads to distal CBD narrowing just above the ampulla of

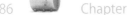

Vater, known as *papillary stenosis*. Patients with papillary stenosis often respond well to biliary sphincterotomy performed via ERCP. HIV cholangiopathy is strongly associated with enteric infection with organisms such as cryptosporidiosis, giardia, etc. Interestingly, treating the underlying infection does not result in improvement in the cholangiopathy itself. We used to see a great number of patients with HIV cholangiopathy, but in the era of modern highly active antiretroviral therapy, we rarely see this complication of HIV anymore. Still, it is important, and you should be aware of it.

- **Drug-induced bile duct disease:** Rarely, patients will develop a chronic inflammatory condition of the bile ducts as a consequence of medications. For example, Adriamycin (doxorubicin), a chemotherapeutic agent, is known to produce cholangiopathy in a small subset of patients who receive it.

- **Immunoglobulin subclass 4 (IgG4)–associated cholangiopathy:** Some patients with an elevated serum IgG4 antibody will develop a chronic inflammatory condition of the bile ducts that can be indistinguishable from PSC on cholangiogram. In contrast to PSC, patients with IgG4-associated cholangiopathy may respond to immunosuppressive agents (steroids, azathioprine, etc). Ampullary biopsies in these patients may stain positive for IgG4 antibodies, and these patients may also develop autoimmune pancreatitis (another IgG4-mediated disease).

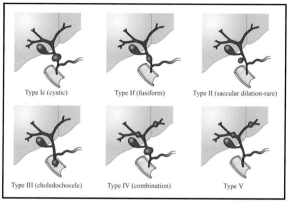

Figure 6-8. A schema showing the common varieties of choledochal cysts.

Biliary Cysts

Biliary cysts can occur anywhere in the biliary tree. Biliary cysts are important because patients who develop them are at increased risk of developing cancer, either within the cyst itself or at another location in the biliary tree. These cancers can be thought of as a form of cholangiocarcinoma or sometimes simply referred to as *biliary adenocarcinomas*.

The following is a somewhat complicated schema for describing congenital biliary cysts (Figure 6-8):

- Type I biliary cysts involve dilation of the CBD. This should not be confused with the more commonly seen dilation of the CBD that occurs after cholecystectomy. Patients with type I biliary cysts are generally treated via surgical resection.
- Type II biliary cysts manifest as diverticula of the extrahepatic biliary tree. These are removed surgically.

- Type III biliary cysts, also referred to as *choledochoceles*, involve the very distal CBD just above the ampulla of Vater. Patients with type III biliary cysts often have an anomalous pancreaticobiliary junction in addition to the cyst itself. Type III biliary cysts have a relatively low risk of undergoing malignant transformation and are often treated via biliary sphincterotomy to promote drainage.

- Type IV biliary cysts involve either multiple cysts of the intra- and extrahepatic ducts or multiple strictures of the extrahepatic ducts only. Surgery can be undertaken in patients with type IV biliary cysts, but this may be difficult given the multifocal nature of the disease.

- Type V biliary cysts are seen in patients with multiple cysts of just the intrahepatic ducts. Patients with type V biliary cysts may have innumerable intrahepatic ductal cysts. This situation is also referred to as *Caroli's disease*. Similar to patients with type IV biliary cysts, surgery in these patients may be problematic due to the extensive nature of the disease.

AMPULLARY DISEASES

The ampulla of Vater typically joins the distal CBD and the pancreatic duct to the second portion of the duodenum. Ampullary diseases are relatively uncommon and few in number but are nonetheless important because they can cause significant disease. It seems appropriate to include them here in the chapter on the bile ducts.

- **Ampullary adenomas:** Ampullary adenomas are adenomatous growths that occur on the ampulla itself. These typically occur on the ampulla of

Vater (also known as the *major papilla*) but can also, although much more rarely, arise on the minor papilla (where the duct of Santorini in the pancreas connects to the duodenum). Ampullary adenomas are typically evaluated via ERCP and endoscopic ultrasound. If ampullary adenomas are not too large and do not manifest deep invasion of the CBD, pancreatic duct, duodenal wall, or pancreatic head, they can be removed endoscopically via ERCP. Some ampullary adenomas, despite their benign nature, are too large to be removed endoscopically and must be removed via surgery, often with a pancreaticoduodenectomy (Whipple procedure). Patients with familial adenomatous polyposis and other polyposis syndromes are at increased risk of developing ampullary adenomas and are often surveyed for them by periodic endoscopy. Ampullary adenomas may be asymptomatic or may produce episodes of pancreatitis and/or jaundice.

- **Ampullary cancer:** If ampullary adenomas are present for a long period of time, they can develop into ampullary cancer, typically adenocarcinomas. Ampullary cancer may closely mimic pancreatic cancer in terms of its presentation (ie, painless jaundice in the setting of weight loss). Similarly, patients with ampullary cancer may develop episodes of acute pancreatitis as part of their presentation. As a general rule, ampullary cancer is treated surgically via a pancreaticoduodenectomy (Whipple procedure). In contrast to pancreatic cancer, which has a dismal long-term prognosis, patients with ampullary cancer can have long-term cures after surgery in the absence of metastases. As you may expect, patients at risk for ampullary adenomas are also at risk for ampullary cancers (Figure 6-9).

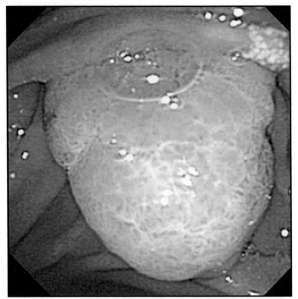

Figure 6-9. An endoscopic image of an advanced ampullary adenoma that contained a focus of ampullary cancer. Compare this image with Figure 3-1 to see the difference between ampullary cancer and a normal ampulla.

BIBLIOGRAPHY

Adler DG, Baron TH, Davila RE, et al; Standards of Practice Committee of American Society for Gastrointestinal Endoscopy. ASGE guideline: the role of ERCP in diseases of the biliary tract and the pancreas. *Gastrointest Endosc.* 2005;62(1):1-8.

Adler DG, Papachristou GI, Taylor LJ, et al. Clinical outcomes in patients with bile leaks treated via ERCP with regard to the timing of ERCP: a large multicenter study. *Gastrointest Endosc.* 2017;85(4):766-772.

Alkhatib AA, Hilden K, Adler DG. Comorbidities, sphincterotomy, and balloon dilation predict post-ERCP adverse events in PSC patients: operator experience is protective. *Dig Dis Sci.* 2011;56(12):3685-3688.

Feurer ME, Hilden K, Adler DG. Primary sclerosing cholangitis and distribution of inflammatory bowel disease. *Clin Gastroenterol Hepatol.* 2012;10(12):1418; author reply 1418-1419.

Gastaca M. Biliary complications after orthotopic liver transplantation: a review of incidence and risk factors. *Transplant Proc.* 2012;44(6):1545-1549.

Nallamothu G, Hilden K, Adler DG. Endoscopic retrograde cholangiopancreatography for non-gastroenterologists: what you need to know. *Hosp Pract (1995).* 2011;39(2):70-80.

Verma D, Kapadia A, Eisen GM, Adler DG. EUS vs MRCP for detection of choledocholithiasis. *Gastrointest Endosc.* 2006;64(2):248-254.

Vitale GC, Davis BR. Evaluation and treatment of biliary leaks after gastrointestinal surgery. *J Gastrointest Surg.* 2011;15(8):1323-1324.

Chapter 7

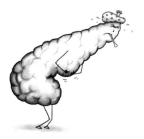

Pancreas

It is fair to say that most people do not even know they have a pancreas. Most people discover that they actually have a pancreas when they or somebody they know develops some form of pancreatic disease, most commonly acute pancreatitis or pancreatic cancer. When this happens, people suddenly realize how important the pancreas is to their daily life and normal health and well-being. In this chapter, we will review the fundamentals of pancreatic function as well as pancreatic disease, both benign and malignant.

Although we commonly think of our stomach as digesting our food, this really is not the case to any large extent. In reality, the stomach serves as a reservoir for swallowed food and begins the process of mechanical digestion via gastric contractions and the effects of

Adler DG. *The Little GI Book: An Easily Digestible Guide to Understanding Gastroenterology, Second Edition* (pp 193-224). © 2020 Taylor & Francis Group.

stomach acid and pepsin on food. It is actually your pancreas that does most of the work of digesting your food via the digestive enzymes the pancreas makes and secretes into the small bowel. Once these enzymes break down food, the small bowel itself absorbs the broken down food into your circulation for your body to use in lots of different ways.

ANATOMY AND PHYSIOLOGY

The pancreas sits behind the stomach and anterior to the spine in the so-called *retroperitoneal space*. The pancreas is described as having a head, body, and tail. The tail is the leftward-most portion of the pancreas, whereas the head is far to the right. The head of the pancreas sits snugly against the second portion of the duodenum, whereas the tail of the pancreas abuts the splenic hilum (where the splenic artery and vein connect to the spleen). The pancreas lies somewhat diagonally, with the tail generally being superior to the head. The portion of the pancreas inferior to the head is referred to as the *uncinate process*, and the portion of the pancreas between the head and the body is referred to as the *genu*. The pancreatic genu is at the site of a bend in the organ, hence the use of the term *genu* (knee) to describe this area. (The act of bending down on one knee is referred to as *genuflection* for this reason.)

Pancreatic tissue is primarily made up of pancreatic acinar cells that make and secrete a variety of digestive enzymes (as well as bicarbonate) into the duodenum where these enzymes mix with food and the work of digestion is accomplished. Running through the pancreatic tissue is the pancreatic ductal system that carries these enzymes and bicarbonate (which are together referred to as *pancreatic juice*) from the acinar cells and into the small bowel. The main pancreatic duct, known as the *duct of Wirsung*, extends all the way from the tail of the pancreas through the body and into the head, where it drains into the second portion of the duodenum via the ampulla of Vater, also known as the *major duodenal papilla*. Of note, the bile ducts also drain into the duodenum via the ampulla of Vater. The main pancreatic duct is generally quite narrow; in a normal adult, the pancreatic duct is approximately 3 mm wide in the head, 2 mm wide in the body, and 1 mm wide in the tail (Figure 7-1). A dilated pancreatic duct is often a sign of pancreatic disease, but we will discuss this more later. A second duct, known as the *duct of Santorini*, communicates with the main pancreatic duct in the head of the gland and drains pancreatic secretions to the duodenum via the minor duodenal papilla. It is worth noting that there are many variations of pancreatic ductal anatomy, some of which are clinically relevant to pancreatic disease.

The acinar cells make 3 types of digestive enzymes: proteases (which break down protein), amylases (which break down carbohydrates), and lipases (which break down fats). The acinar cells secrete these enzymes, along with bicarbonate, into the pancreatic ducts in inactive forms known as *zymogens*. When they leave the pancreas and are exposed to the physiologic milieu of the duodenum, these inactive enzyme forms become fully functional and can begin to digest food. The enzymes are secreted in an inactive form as a safety mechanism; if the enzymes were active as soon as they were manufactured in the pancreas, there would be nothing to stop these digestive enzymes from digesting the pancreas itself!

In addition to acinar cells, the pancreas also contains groups of cells known as *islets of Langerhans*. These islets, which are dispersed throughout the entire pancreas, produce a variety of hormones. The most important of these hormones include glucagon (which is secreted by alpha cells) and insulin (which is secreted by beta cells). Glucagon functions to increase serum blood glucose

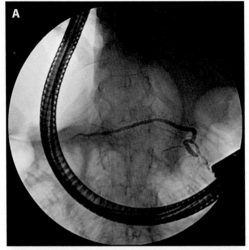

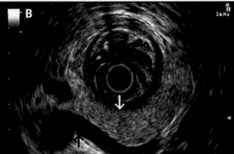

Figure 7-1. (A) A normal pancreatogram as seen via endoscopic retrograde cholangiopancreatography (ERCP) with tapering of the duct toward the tail, smooth walls, and normal side branches. (B) A normal pancreatic genu and body as seen via endoscopic ultrasound (EUS). The normal, homogeneous pancreas is in the center of the image (white arrow). The splenic vein is seen below and alongside the pancreas and merges with the portal vein on the left of the image (black arrow).

levels, whereas insulin reduces serum glucose levels. These and other hormones from the islet cells are released directly into the systemic circulation and are not passed into the duodenum via ducts. The adjustment of blood glucose levels is closely tied to digestive function, so it makes sense that the pancreas should have both endocrine (active agents released into the bloodstream) and exocrine (active agents released into the ducts and bowel) function.

ACUTE PANCREATITIS

Acute pancreatitis is the most commonly encountered pancreatic disease. As the name suggests, acute pancreatitis involves inflammation of the pancreas that is often rapid in onset. Acute pancreatitis has a classic clinical presentation wherein patients develop epigastric and/or right upper quadrant pain that radiates to their back. This pain can be very severe. Acute pancreatitis comes with an accompanying rise in pancreatic blood tests, most commonly the serum amylase and lipase levels. Many patients with acute pancreatitis also experience severe nausea and vomiting.

Acute pancreatitis can be clinically mild, moderate, or severe. The severity of the symptoms does not correlate well to the actual severity of the pancreatitis attack (ie, some of the people who feel the worst can have just mild pancreatitis that is extremely painful). Conversely, I have seen patients with severe necrotizing pancreatitis who have comparatively less pain and objectively look better. Most patients with mild pancreatitis will recover quickly when treated with conservative measures, such as aggressive hydration and nothing by mouth (also known as *nil per os*) status. Patients with moderate or severe pancreatitis can develop complications, including peripancreatic fluid collections referred to as *pseudocysts*, pancreatic abscesses, pancreatic ductal injuries, and pancreatic

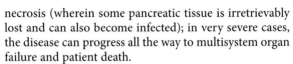

necrosis (wherein some pancreatic tissue is irretrievably lost and can also become infected); in very severe cases, the disease can progress all the way to multisystem organ failure and patient death.

Most patients who develop acute pancreatitis develop so-called *interstitial pancreatitis*. In these patients, the pancreas is edematous and swollen, and there is generally an absence of hemorrhage. Most patients with interstitial pancreatitis recover normal pancreatic structure and function when the episode of pancreatitis resolves. More severe forms of acute pancreatitis include hemorrhagic pancreatitis and/or necrotizing pancreatitis as mentioned previously. Patients with hemorrhagic and/or necrotizing pancreatitis are at a much higher risk of complications and dying.

Pathophysiology

Although the exact mechanism by which acute pancreatitis occurs remains controversial, most data suggest that the premature activation of pancreatic zymogens (while these enzymes are still within the pancreas) leads to acute pancreatitis. Acute pancreatitis can occur in patients with pancreatic ductal obstruction, although many patients with pancreatitis will have no evidence of ductal obstruction. In some patients, diminished pancreatic blood flow (known as *ischemia*) may play a role, but this is not universally seen. Premature activation of pancreatic enzymes within the pancreas results in autodigestion of the pancreas itself, which can lead to further inflammation, vascular damage, and the release of proinflammatory mediators known as *cytokines*. All of these factors likely play a role in establishing a case of acute pancreatitis.

Etiology

The search for causes of acute pancreatitis has been extensive and fruitful, and many causative factors have been identified over the years. The following is a list of some of the most common causes of pancreatitis, but in up to 15% of patients, no cause will ever be identified.

- Gallstones are the most common cause of pancreatitis. Small stones can escape the gallbladder via transiting the cystic duct and getting into the common bile duct. The distal common bile duct joins the pancreatic duct in the head of the pancreas at the level of the ampulla of Vater, and bile duct stones can obstruct the pancreatic duct and start the cycle of events that leads to an episode of acute pancreatitis.

- Alcohol is commonly implicated in patients with acute pancreatitis, and many patients will develop pancreatitis after an episode of heavy drinking, although some will develop an episode of pancreatitis in the setting of modest alcohol consumption.

- Trauma, especially in children, is another common cause of acute pancreatitis. In adults, a fall or a motor vehicle accident (wherein the patient's upper abdomen impacts the steering wheel) is a typically encountered story, whereas in children a fall off of a bicycle (with an associated impact against the handlebars) is what you might hear.

- Medications are often implicated in patients who develop acute pancreatitis but who have no history of gallstones, alcohol use, or trauma. The list of medications that have an association with acute pancreatitis is long, but some commonly encountered agents with relatively strong associations include thiazide diuretics, loop diuretics, azathioprine, 6-mercaptopurine, asparaginase, selective serotonin reuptake inhibitor antidepressants,

angiotensin-converting enzyme inhibitors, val-
proic acid, and estrogens. The full list of medications with an association with acute pancreatitis
is quite extensive, and if you suspect a patient may
have drug-induced pancreatitis, you should investigate each of his or her medications individually.

- Hypercalcemia, often due to primary or secondary
hyperparathyroidism or bony metastases, can lead
to acute pancreatitis.

- Hypertriglyceridemia, often with levels above
500 mg/dL, is another common cause of acute pancreatitis and should be treated with lipid-lowering
agents when found.

- Iatrogenic pancreatitis is most typically seen in
patients after undergoing ERCP (referred to as
post-ERCP pancreatitis) but can occur after other
procedures as well.

- Genetic causes should be suspected in young
patients with no other obvious etiologies, especially if there is a family history of other similar
events. Genetic tests can be performed via simple
blood tests. It is worth remembering that genetic
testing can sometimes lead to results that are difficult to interpret and may be upsetting to patients.
Also, genetic testing can be expensive and may not
be covered by insurance. If you are going to test
patients for hereditary pancreatitis, you need to
check for 3 main genetic abnormalities:

  ○ **Cystic fibrosis:** Abnormalities in the cystic
  fibrosis gene (known as *CFTR*) can commonly
  lead to pancreatitis, both acute and eventually chronic pancreatitis. Often, patients with
  CFTR mutations do not have classic cystic
  fibrosis but rather have other mutations in the
  CFTR gene that lead to pancreatitis. Be aware
  that if you check a patient for cystic fibrosis

mutations, you may discover that he or she has a mutation that is not associated with either cystic fibrosis disease or pancreatitis. It is often hard to know what to do with these types of results.

○ *Serine protease inhibitor Kazal-type 1 (SPINK): SPINK* is also sometimes referred to as *SPINK1*. Patients with *SPINK* mutations are at increased risk of developing pancreatitis because of autoactivation of pancreatic enzymes that the body cannot shut off.

○ *PRSS1:* This gene codes for a type of enzyme that breaks down proteins (a protease) known as *trypsinogen*. Trypsinogen is converted to trypsin, the active form of the enzyme. People with *PRSS1* mutations produce a form of trypsin that is difficult to inactivate or may prematurely inactivate, leading to autodigestion of the pancreas and pancreatitis.

Diagnosis

The typical clinical presentation of a patient with acute pancreatitis includes epigastric abdominal pain, which can be severe (often radiating to the back), as well as nausea and vomiting. The pain is usually constant and does not go away with changes in position. The pain is often more severe when the patient leans back and may lessen if the patient leans forward. Patients may be pale and distressed and have other symptoms including a distended abdomen, jaundice, fevers, and tachycardia. Grey Turner's sign (flank bruising, which can be unilateral or bilateral) or Cullen's sign (bruising surrounding the navel) may be present. Patients with more severe pancreatitis may be clinically unstable with hypotension or shock due to volume depletion and/or sepsis.

To diagnose a patient with acute pancreatitis, you generally need to have at least 2 out of the 3 following findings: serum amylase and lipase levels greater than 3 times above the upper limit of normal, a clinical picture similar to that described previously with typical epigastric abdominal pain, and imaging features consistent with pancreatitis on computed tomography (CT) scanning or magnetic resonance imaging (MRI). Note that you only need 2 of these 3 features; what this really means is that if the patient has a strong clinical presentation and lab work suggestive of acute pancreatitis, you do not necessarily require imaging to confirm the diagnosis.

Other findings that are often seen in patients with acute pancreatitis include dehydration and decreased urine output, hypotension, a rise in the patient's hematocrit secondary to hemoconcentration, acute respiratory distress syndrome/respiratory failure, metabolic acidosis, renal failure, and fluctuation in serum calcium levels.

Patients with mild acute pancreatitis can often be managed in a general medicine inpatient setting. Patients with severe pancreatitis often need intensive care unit–level care.

Treatment

Mild Pancreatitis

Most patients who develop pancreatitis will have the mild form of the disease, sometimes referred to as *interstitial pancreatitis*. In these patients, the pancreas is swollen and inflamed, but when the inflammation goes away, the pancreas returns to normal in terms of both structure and function. Patients with mild pancreatitis may feel horrible and have severe pain, but they tend to recover in short order, typically 2 to 4 days.

Patients with mild pancreatitis should be treated with adequate IV fluid resuscitation, analgesic pain medication as needed (usually in the form of narcotics), and nothing by mouth status. I cannot state strongly enough how important IV hydration of these patients is. The most common mistake clinicians make when treating patients with acute pancreatitis is underhydrating them. Adequate hydration can help prevent injury to other organs (ie, the kidneys) and often helps patients to improve clinically more quickly. Patients can generally be fed when they are hungry but should advance their diet slowly from clear liquids to a normal diet over the course of several days.

If the patient has mild pancreatitis, the treatment is often straightforward, and the patient usually recovers without incident. It is always important to make sure that an etiology for the episode is identified if at all possible (ie, if the patient has gallstone pancreatitis, the patient may need an evaluation for ERCP to remove common bile duct stones and/or a cholecystectomy to prevent future episodes of pancreatitis). If the patient is felt to have taken an offending medication, this agent should be stopped and a suitable alternative selected.

Severe Pancreatitis

In contrast to patients with mild pancreatitis, patients with severe pancreatitis rarely recover quickly and may have a prolonged hospitalization. These patients are typically very ill, and many require treatment in an intensive care unit. Patients with severe pancreatitis often develop intra-abdominal fluid collections and inflammatory cysts known as *pancreatic pseudocysts*. They may even have part of their pancreas die due to severe inflammation and loss of blood flow; this is termed *pancreatic necrosis*. Patients can also often develop extrapancreatic side effects of the disease, including the development of respiratory, renal, or circulatory compromise or failure. Usually, these patients need many doctors to care for them, including intensive care physicians, gastroenterologists, surgeons, interventional radiologists, etc.

Just as in patients with mild pancreatitis, patients with severe pancreatitis need adequate pain management and IV fluid replacement. Urine output should be closely monitored to watch for the development of renal failure, which would require hemodialysis.

Most acute fluid collections in the abdomen and/or pseudocysts are simply observed unless they develop complications that would warrant some form of interventional procedure. These fluid collections or pseudocysts can become infected (which can be a medical and/or surgical emergency) or can become so large that they compress other organs to the point that those organs do not function properly. It is not uncommon for pseudocysts to compress the stomach or bowel to the point that the cysts need to be drained to allow the gut to begin to function normally again. If fluid collections or pseudocysts need to be drained, surgical, endoscopic, or percutaneous options exist and are usually selected depending on local expertise.

As with mild pancreatitis, patients with severe acute pancreatitis are usually not fed anything for at least 48 hours after diagnosis. If pancreatic necrosis is seen, enteral feeding (ie, using the gut as opposed to IV feeding) using a nasoenteric tube is often performed. In these patients, a narrow feeding tube is inserted into the patient's nose and advanced so that the distal tip of the tube is placed beyond the ligament of Treitz (at which point, the tube is in the distal duodenum/proximal jejunum). Food inserted into the small bowel at this point will not stimulate the pancreas and is safe to use.

The idea of feeding patients with severe pancreatitis seems counterintuitive (given that you do not feed patients with mild pancreatitis at all!), but it actually makes sense. Feeding patients with severe pancreatitis via a feeding tube into the small bowel at a point where the pancreas is functionally "blind" to the food allows the patient's bowels to work normally and likely helps reduce the risk of the patient developing an infection of the pancreas itself. If the patient has necrosis and it becomes infected, the risk of the patient dying becomes significant.

Tube feeding in this manner is often performed to reduce the risk of bacterial translocation from the gut to the necrotic pancreas. Having the gut work in a normal fashion will also potentially improve intestinal wall integrity as well. I should state that this approach, although widespread, is somewhat controversial, and different opinions exist regarding feeding patients with severe pancreatitis.

Other options for feeding patients with severe acute pancreatitis include IV feeding in the form of total parenteral nutrition (TPN). This allows a patient to get all of his or her calories, nutrients, vitamins, and minerals in a single IV solution given over the course of a day. If TPN is used, the patient can be reintroduced to food at a later time when he or she is more stable clinically.

TPN was once the standard treatment in patients with severe acute pancreatitis, but some studies have shown that it has been associated with increased costs, length of hospital stay, and complications. Others say that TPN may increase overall mortality rates and raise the risk of developing systemic and local infections. Still, despite these risks, TPN is the best option for providing nutrition in some patients.

Patients who develop pancreatic necrosis (dead pancreas) must be carefully monitored for the development of infected pancreatic necrosis. Patients with infected pancreatic necrosis can decompensate and die quickly without proper treatment. Patients with extensive pancreatic necrosis are at a higher risk of infection when compared with those with only a small area of necrosis. Infected pancreatic necrosis used to be commonly treated with surgical debridement, although this has been almost completely replaced via endoscopic debridement. (See Chapter 8 for a more in-depth description of endoscopic drainage and debridement of pancreatic pseudocysts and necrosis.) In some cases, antibiotics alone may be all that is required to treat patients with infected pancreatic necrosis.

Patients with infected pancreatic necrosis may need several operations and/or other drainage procedures to completely remove all of the dead and infected tissue. These patients, if they survive, may become lifelong diabetics given the loss of the insulin-producing islets of Langerhans.

The use of antibiotics in patients with confirmed pancreatic necrosis (in an attempt to avoid infection of the dead pancreatic tissue) is common but nonetheless remains controversial. Different research studies have shown conflicting results as to whether this idea (which seems to make sense on the surface) is really helpful or not. Antibiotics such as imipenem, meropenem, and the fluoroquinolones have a high degree of pancreatic penetrance and are commonly used to try to "sterilize" necrotic pancreatic tissue. Most physicians who use antibiotics in this situation recommend a 14- to 21-day course.

IMAGING STUDIES IN PANCREATITIS

Standard X-Rays

On abdominal x-rays, the presence of calcifications (calcium deposits in the pancreas) may suggest an underlying diagnosis of chronic pancreatitis. Another finding that may be seen on an abdominal x-ray in pancreatitis is the so-called *sentinel loop*, which represents a dilated segment of small intestine or colon that is not contracting properly (known as an *ileus*). Rarely, calcified gallstones in the gallbladder or common bile duct can be seen (suggesting gallstone pancreatitis as a cause of the disease).

Right Upper Quadrant Transabdominal Ultrasound

A hyperechoic (bright) and enlarged pancreas is often seen on transabdominal ultrasound in patients with acute pancreatitis, although the pancreas itself may be seen poorly overall on this study. Overlying bowel gas tends to obscure the pancreas. Still, right upper quadrant ultrasound is often very helpful in patients with pancreatitis because it gives us a lot of information about the gallbladder and the bile ducts in patients with suspected gallstone pancreatitis. Right upper quadrant ultrasound can identify stones in the gallbladder and evidence of acute or chronic cholecystis, including gallbladder wall thickening and/or pericholecystic fluid (cholecystitis often occurs at the same time as gallstone pancreatitis). Right upper quadrant ultrasound can also look at the common bile duct for dilation (which may be present if there is an obstructing common bile duct stone). In some cases, this study can actually see a stone in the common bile duct, but this is the exception and not the rule in my experience. A right upper quadrant ultrasound does not provide much information regarding the extent of pancreatic inflammation or the presence or absence of pancreatic necrosis.

Computed Tomography Scans

CT scans, with intravenous (IV) contrast if the patient has been adequately hydrated, are very helpful studies in patients with pancreatitis, especially if you think the patient may have a more severe form of the disease. With a good-quality CT scan, the entire pancreas can be seen, and any areas of necrosis and/or inflammatory fluid collections (pseudocysts) can be identified. CT scans are less than ideal studies for looking at the gallbladder and common bile duct but can often still provide useful information about these structures.

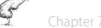
Magnetic Resonance Imaging Scans

A good-quality MRI of the abdomen can provide you with a wealth of information in patients with pancreatitis. MRI is highly effective at identifying fluid collections and pancreatic necrosis, but the great advantage of MRI is that a special type of MRI, known as *magnetic resonance cholangiopancreatography* (MRCP), can provide extremely detailed views of the bile ducts to look for common bile duct stones. MRCP can also give you a lot of information about the gallbladder, such as whether or not there are gallbladder stones or inflammation. Small hospitals may still not have access to MRI or may not be able to perform MRCP even if they have an MRI machine.

Endoscopic Ultrasound

EUS is commonly performed to evaluate the common bile duct for the presence of stones that may require removal (usually via ERCP). EUS is of relatively little value with regard to inspecting the pancreas during an episode of pancreatitis because the inflammation often precludes a detailed evaluation of the gland. If stones are seen during an EUS examination, ERCP is usually indicated. EUS and MRI/MRCP are equally good at detecting common bile duct stones.

CHRONIC PANCREATITIS

Despite the similarity in name, chronic pancreatitis refers to a very different disease than acute pancreatitis. Acute pancreatitis generally refers to an acute inflammatory process that, when it subsides, often returns the pancreas to its baseline state of structure and function. In contrast, chronic pancreatitis refers to a disease in which there has been permanent scarring and injury to the pancreas with alteration in the baseline structure and function of the gland.

Similarly, most patients with acute pancreatitis require inpatient hospitalization. Most patients with chronic pancreatitis are treated as outpatients and are only admitted to the hospital for severe flares of their disease. Acute pancreatitis is often caused by a focal insult to the gland (gallstone pancreatitis, a reaction to medication, etc), whereas chronic pancreatitis is generally caused by chronic insults to the gland that are ongoing over a long period of time. In patients with chronic pancreatitis, the pancreas becomes the setting for alternating waves of inflammation and fibrosis, which ultimately leave the gland atrophic, scarred, and with the loss of overall exocrine and endocrine function. The pancreatic duct over time may dilate and develop strictures, stones, or both (Figure 7-2).

Etiology

- **Alcohol use:** Alcohol use is the overwhelmingly most common cause of chronic pancreatitis worldwide. I have listed it here as the number one cause of chronic pancreatitis, but I often like to joke with my students that it is actually the number 1, 2, and 3 causes of the disease. As a rule, one must consume alcohol on a regular basis at a fairly high level for a number of years to cause chronic pancreatitis. However, this does vary significantly between patients. Some patients can consume alcohol for many years and only develop mild chronic pancreatitis or no chronic pancreatitis at all, whereas other patients may have a brief period (3 to 5 years) during which they consumed alcohol very heavily and go on to develop severe chronic pancreatitis.

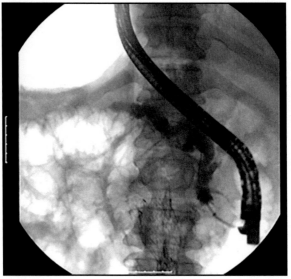

Figure 7-2. An abnormal pancreatogram as seen via ERCP in a patient with chronic pancreatitis. The duct is massively dilated, tortuous in contour, and has dilated and irregular side branches. Compare with Figure 7-1A (a normal pancreatogram) to highlight the differences.

- **Genetic causes:** Several inherited genetic disorders can lead to chronic pancreatitis. Cystic fibrosis is the genetic disease that is most commonly linked to chronic pancreatitis. Patients with classic cystic fibrosis often develop a fatty atrophic pancreas. In contrast, when patients with chronic pancreatitis are evaluated, many of them have mutations in the cystic fibrosis gene that are not classically associated with florid cystic fibrosis (ie, pulmonary symptoms). There are also other genetic causes of chronic pancreatitis that can be tested for; these typically involve errors in the genes of the pancreatic enzyme that lead to early activation or inappropriate activation of the enzymes within the pancreas.

- **Autoimmune pancreatitis:** Autoimmune pancreatitis, as the name suggests, reflects an autoimmune attack on the pancreas by the patient's own immune system. Autoimmune pancreatitis can present in both acute and chronic forms and is typically associated with an elevated serum immunoglobulin G subclass 4. Autoimmune pancreatitis often leads to extrahepatic biliary strictures (as the distal common bile duct runs through the head of the pancreas, the common bile duct becomes compressed and/or obstructed when the surrounding pancreas swells) and pancreatic duct strictures. Autoimmune pancreatitis is often treated with steroids or other immunosuppressants. Autoimmune pancreatitis can closely mimic pancreatic cancer and is sometimes treated surgically if the true diagnosis is not identified.

- **Tropical pancreatitis:** Tropical pancreatitis refers to a form of chronic pancreatitis that is often seen in tropical Asia, India, and parts of Africa. The cause of tropical pancreatitis is poorly understood, and the disease can develop even in small children.

- **Pancreatic trauma:** Pancreatic trauma can lead to chronic pancreatic duct injury and obstruction, which, if untreated, can lead to chronic pancreatitis.

- Other causes for chronic pancreatitis include untreated hyperparathyroidism (which can lead to chronic hypercalcemia), congenital abnormalities of the pancreatic duct, and so-called *idiopathic chronic pancreatitis* in which patients have no clear cause for the disease but have clinical and imaging findings consistent with chronic pancreatitis.

Symptoms

- **Pain:** The most common symptom of chronic pancreatitis is abdominal pain. The pain is classically epigastric with radiation to the back that is made worse by eating. Patients may have long periods where they have little to no pain followed by weeks to months of severe pain. Many patients with chronic pancreatitis will attempt to self-medicate using alcohol, which, as you would expect, only makes things worse.

- **Diabetes:** Chronic pancreatitis causes pancreatic atrophy with loss of overall pancreatic tissue over time. This includes the islets of Langerhans. As patients lose insulin-producing cells over time, they often develop diabetes.

- **Malabsorption and diarrhea:** Patients with chronic pancreatitis often eventually lose their ability to secrete enough pancreatic enzymes into the duodenum. This can occur either due to general loss of pancreatic tissue so that inadequate enzymes and bicarbonate can be produced in the first place or as a consequence of pancreatic ductal obstruction. If the pancreatic duct is obstructed, any bicarbonate and pancreatic enzymes manufactured in the pancreas may be unable to reach the duodenum at all. Patients with chronic pancreatitis and malabsorptive diarrhea typically have greasy foul-smelling stools known as *steatorrhea*. These patients typically develop chronic weight loss as well.

- **Fat-soluble vitamin deficiency:** Fat-soluble vitamin deficiencies are common in patients with chronic pancreatitis. This is a key side effect of their overall malabsorptive state. Vitamins A, D, E, and K are the fat-soluble vitamins, and patients may develop night blindness, osteoporosis, easy bruisability, and other symptoms.

- **Strictures of the pancreatic ducts and common bile duct:** Pancreatic duct strictures often develop as a consequence of inflammation and can promote an overall worsening of the disease in patients with chronic pancreatitis (ie, inflammation gives rise to a stricture, the gland becomes obstructed, enzymes activate in the blocked duct, which gives rise to more inflammation, which can lead to more strictures, and so on). Patients with inflammation in the pancreatic head often develop distal bile duct strictures as well. In these patients, the bile duct was an innocent bystander of sorts that was just passing through the pancreas on its way to the ampulla of Vater, but the surrounding inflammation caused extrinsic compression, which can lead to jaundice.

- **Pancreatic duct stones:** Inflammation and strictures in the pancreatic ducts can lead to the formation of pancreatic duct stones. These can range from simple to very difficult to remove endoscopically. Some patients require very aggressive therapy, including surgery, to remove pancreatic duct stones and decompress the pancreatic duct.

- **Increased risk of pancreatic adenocarcinoma:** Although an increased risk of pancreatic cancer is not really a symptom of chronic pancreatitis per se, it is worth commenting on. Chronic pancreatitis from any cause increases a patient's lifetime risk of developing pancreatic cancer, probably as a consequence of chronic inflammation. Many of the symptoms of chronic pancreatitis overlap with that of pancreatic cancer, and it can often be difficult to identify pancreatic cancer in a patient with chronic pancreatitis.

Treatment

The treatment of chronic pancreatitis is aimed at removing inciting factors and treating symptoms.

- Alcohol abstinence is critical in most patients but in practice is very hard to achieve. Tobacco cessation is also vital in these patients because smoking/chewing is associated with an increased risk of developing pancreatic cancer. It should be stressed that if you can get the patient to stop drinking, he or she may have resolution of pain without the addition of any medications.

- Pain management via medications or nerve blocks (known as *celiac blocks*) is often undertaken. Pain management in these patients can be tricky because many are alcoholics and/or substance abusers, and physicians are often hesitant to prescribe narcotic medications to patients with a history of substance abuse. A non-narcotic treatment for painful chronic pancreatitis is pregabalin, which some patients find helpful.

- Enzyme supplementation via the use of orally administered exogenous pancreatic enzymes can be very successful at treating steatorrhea/malabsorptive diarrhea. Some patients and physicians believe that the use of pancreatic enzyme supplements can also help to improve chronic pain in these patients, but this is very controversial.

- Pancreatic duct stones and strictures can be treated via endoscopic and/or surgical means in an attempt to decompress the pancreatic duct and reduce pain as well.

- Biliary strictures secondary to chronic pancreatitis are usually treated via ERCP with the placement of biliary stents. In some patients, these biliary strictures can become intractable and require the creation of a surgical biliary bypass.

- Fat-soluble vitamin replacement (often in the context of taking a generic multivitamin) is helpful because many of these patients have become vitamin deficient due to prolonged malabsorption and malnutrition.

- Pancreatic cancer screening is warranted in these patients given their high risk of developing pancreatic cancer but is costly and may not reduce the risk of dying from pancreatic cancer if it develops. Furthermore, there are no universally agreed-on surveillance regimens.

- Surgery is an option for patients with chronic pancreatitis. This is a somewhat extreme option that most patients try to avoid. Options for surgery in patients with chronic pancreatitis include the following:

  ◦ Decompressive surgeries that aim to relieve the pressure on an obstructed pancreatic duct

  ◦ Resections that aim to remove focal areas of bad chronic pancreatitis (ie, a distal pancreatectomy in someone with a particularly inflamed pancreatic tail or a pancreaticoduodenectomy in someone with a focally inflamed pancreatic head)

  ◦ Total pancreatectomy in patients with severe, end-stage chronic pancreatitis and debilitating pain or other severe symptoms. If a pancreatectomy is done in isolation, that patient will become an insulin-dependent diabetic. At some centers, the insulin-producing islet cells are removed from the explanted pancreas and put back into the patient to prevent diabetes, a procedure known as *total pancreatectomy with islet cell autotransplantation.*

SOLID PANCREATIC TUMORS

Pancreatic Adenocarcinoma

Pancreatic adenocarcinoma (often simply termed *pancreatic cancer*) is the most common solid tumor of the pancreas. Although a relatively rare form of cancer, pancreatic cancer is a leading cause of cancer-related death because most patients who are diagnosed with the disease will die of it. Pancreatic cancer often presents in advanced stages, when few viable treatment options are effective. Patients with early pancreatic cancer at the time of diagnosis tend to do the best, but they are relatively few in number because early pancreatic cancer is often asymptomatic. Patients with pancreatic cancer in the head of the gland often have associated obstruction of the bile ducts (which leads to jaundice) and can also develop obstruction of the duodenum (which leads to gastric outlet obstruction). Both of these problems can be treated with endoscopic stents.

Pancreatic cancer can sometimes be treated via surgery. If the tumor does not invade the aorta (AO), celiac artery (CA), or superior mesenteric artery (SMA) and there is no evidence of metastases, patients may undergo surgery (Figure 7-3). Tumors that involve the superior mesenteric vein or portal vein are considered to be "borderline resectable" and may warrant preoperative chemotherapy and/or radiation therapy. These patients may require venous reconstruction during surgery. Tumors that involve just the splenic artery (eg, those in the tail) can usually be removed.

Tumors in the head are treated by a pancreaticoduodenectomy (sometimes referred to as a *Whipple procedure*, which usually involves the removal of the head of the pancreas, the first and second portion of the duodenum, part of the stomach, and the gallbladder), and tumors in the body and tail may be treated by a distal pancreatectomy

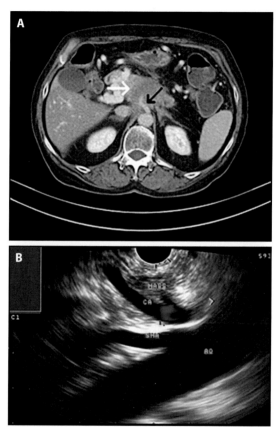

Figure 7-3. (A) A CT scan of a solid pancreatic mass (white arrow) that encases the CA (black arrow). Thus, this patient has unresectable pancreatic cancer. (B) An EUS image of the same patient as in A showing the mass encasing the CA as it arises from the AO from a side view. The SMA is free of tumor.

(which often includes a splenectomy). Patients with metastases or arterial involvement are considered inoperable. Chemotherapy and radiation therapy are also often used to treat pancreatic cancer, both in the preoperative (neoadjuvant) and postoperative (adjuvant) settings.

Some risk factors for pancreatic cancer include the following:

- Age greater than 60 years
- Chronic pancreatitis of any cause
- Obesity
- History of a partial gastrectomy or (maybe) cholecystectomy
- Tobacco use
- Hereditary pancreatitis (usually *PRSS1* gene mutations)
- *CDKN2A*, *BRCA1*, and *BRCA2* gene mutations
- Peutz-Jeghers syndrome
- Lynch syndrome (a colonic polyposis syndrome)
- Ataxia telangiectasia

Neuroendocrine Tumors of the Pancreas

Neuroendocrine tumors are much less common solid tumors of the pancreas but are important to know about because they may have a better prognosis than pancreatic adenocarcinoma if diagnosed and treated early. Neuroendocrine tumors are often known for secreting hormones that are biologically active. These hormones produce symptoms that may help suggest the presence of the tumor itself and lead to an earlier diagnosis. Although commonly arising in the pancreas, some of these tumors can also arise in other locations, such as the duodenum, liver, or lungs. Some types of neuroendocrine tumors include the following:

- **Nonfunctioning neuroendocrine tumors:** These are neuroendocrine tumors that produce no hormones but can still metastasize to other organs and are a form of cancer.

- **Insulinomas:** These tumors can produce excessive insulin resulting in hypoglycemia, syncope (fainting episodes), confusion, palpitations, or tremulousness. Insulinomas can be very small and difficult to detect on scans, although EUS can often detect insulinomas.

- **Glucagonomas:** These tumors produce the hormone glucagon. Patients with glucagonomas can develop hyperglycemia, diabetes, diarrhea, blood clots, and a particular rash called *necrolytic migratory erythema*. Necrolytic migratory erythema often involves the groin/thighs, but it can also affect the face or the arms and legs. The rash produces red plaques or papules.

- **VIPomas:** These tumors produce vasoactive intestinal polypeptide (VIP). Patients with VIPomas often present with profound watery diarrhea and associated electrolyte disorders.

- **Gastrinomas:** Gastrinomas overproduce the hormone gastrin, which stimulates the stomach to produce acid. Patients with gastrinomas frequently develop difficult-to-treat gastric and duodenal ulcers. Patients in this situation are said to have Zollinger-Ellison syndrome.

- **Somatostatinomas:** These tumors overproduce the hormone somatostatin, which is classically thought of as a gut-inhibitory hormone. Patients with somatostatinomas will often develop diarrhea, malabsorption, diabetes (from insulin inhibition), and gallbladder stones (from cholecystokinin inhibition), among other symptoms.

- Other, rare neuroendocrine tumors include tumors that release agents such as parathyroid hormone, adrenocorticotropic hormone, calcitonin, and growth hormone (among others).

Cystic Lesions of the Pancreas

Cystic lesions of the pancreas are a common finding—we see these all the time. These may be discovered incidentally during the evaluation of other symptoms (ie, a renal protocol CT scan to investigate kidney stones reveals a pancreatic cyst) or may be found during an investigation of abdominal pain or pancreatitis.

Pancreatic cysts can be of no malignant potential, premalignant, or frankly malignant. The management of pancreatic cysts is often difficult because many patients have no symptoms, some lesions may have low malignant potential, and the surgeries to remove these lesions are often very involved. Thus, many of these lesions are simply observed rather than resected. As a general rule of thumb, cysts containing serous (watery) fluid are more likely to be benign, whereas cysts containing mucus (also known as *mucinous cysts*) are more likely to be premalignant or frankly malignant.

The differential diagnosis of a pancreatic cyst includes the following:

- **Simple cysts:** These are usually small, unilocular serous cysts that are lined by benign epithelium. These are often observed without surgery.

- **Pseudocysts:** These are inflammatory cysts that usually form due to a prior episode of pancreatitis. They may contain debris, old blood, or other contents. They are called *pseudocysts* because they have no true epithelial lining. These can be

asymptomatic or may require drainage via percutaneous, endoscopic, or surgical means (Figure 7-4).

- **Serous cystadenomas:** These lesions often appear
  as a collection of small to large cysts that often have
  an associated central scar. These cysts are thought
  to have little to no malignant potential.

- **Mucinous cystadenomas:** As the name implies,
  these are mucin-containing cysts. These do have
  malignant potential and can turn into mucinous
  cystadenocarcinomas (Figure 7-5).

- **Intraductal papillary mucinous neoplasms
  (IPMNs):** These are another type of mucin-
  producing tumor that can involve the main pancreatic duct or pancreatic duct side branches.
  IPMNs have a real potential for malignant transformation, and those that involve the main duct
  are often resected. Small side-branch IPMNs can
  be observed periodically via CT or MRI scans for
  changes that would warrant surgery.

- **Solid pseudopapillary tumors of the pancreas:**
  These lesions can present as a mixed solid/cystic
  tumor that can range in size from subcentimeter
  lesions to large macroscopic lesions greater than
  10 cm in size. These are often seen in young female
  patients and are often resected because they can
  cause abdominal pain.

Cystic lesions of the pancreas are often identified via
imaging studies such as CT or MRI scans. Many patients
with a pancreatic cyst will then be referred to undergo
an EUS with fine-needle aspiration of the cyst. The aspirated fluid is then sent for analysis. Common fluid analysis includes an evaluation for amylase and lipase levels
as well as measurement of the tumor marker known
as *carcinoembryonic antigen*. The fluid is also checked

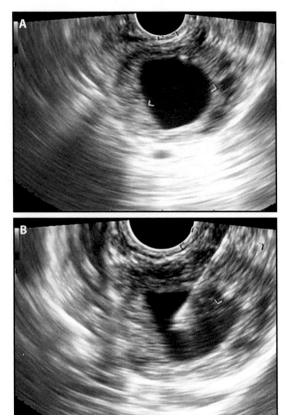

Figure 7-4. (A) A thick-walled pseudocyst seen on EUS in a patient with a history of pancreatitis. (B) The same patient as seen in A now undergoing EUS-guided fine-needle aspiration of the lesion.

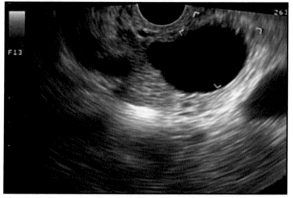

Figure 7-5. A unilocular cystic lesion in the pancreas as seen on EUS. Fine-needle aspiration revealed a mucinous cystadenoma. The patient underwent surgical resection.

for mucin. DNA analysis can also be undertaken if so desired to further assess the potential for malignancy or future malignant transformation. Tumors with a high carcinoembryonic antigen level and the presence of mucin are often treated surgically.

Whether a patient with a potentially malignant pancreatic cystic lesion should undergo surgery is a common dilemma for both doctors and patients because the risks of the lesion need to be weighed against the risks of the surgery to remove it (there is no such thing as "small" pancreatic surgery) and the patient's overall health and life expectancy.

BIBLIOGRAPHY

Adler DG. Single-operator experience with a 20-mm diameter lumen apposing metal stent to treat patients with large pancreatic fluid collections from pancreatic necrosis. *Endosc Ultrasound*. 2018;7(6):422-423.

Adler DG. Primary endoscopic therapy should be preferred over surgery for patients with infected pancreatic necrosis. *Gastroenterology*. 2018;154(5):1541-1542.

Adler DG. Surgery versus endoscopy for patients with infected pancreatic necrosis. *Lancet*. 2018;391(10115):6-8.

Adler DG, Shah J, Nieto J, et al. Placement of lumen-apposing metal stents to drain pseudocysts and walled-off pancreatic necrosis can be safely performed on an outpatient basis: a multicenter study. *Endosc Ultrasound*. 2019;8(1):36-42.

Goodman AJ, Gress FG. The endoscopic management of pain in chronic pancreatitis. *Gastroenterol Res Pract*. 2012;2012:860879.

Sugumar A, Chari ST. Autoimmune pancreatitis. *J Gastroenterol Hepatol*. 2011;26(9):1368-1373.

Vanwoerkom R, Adler DG. Acute pancreatitis: review and clinical update. *Hosp Physician*. 2009;45(1):9-19.

van Brunschot S, van Grinsven J, van Santvoort HC, et al; Dutch Pancreatitis Study Group. Endoscopic or surgical step-up approach for infected necrotising pancreatitis: a multicenter randomised trial. *Lancet*. 2018;391(10115):51-58.

Verma D, Kapadia A, Eisen GM, Adler DG. EUS vs MRCP for detection of choledocholithiasis. *Gastrointest Endosc*. 2006;64(2):248-254.

Chapter 8

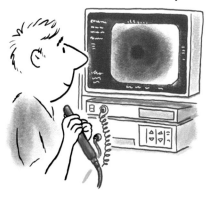

Endoscopy

Although all gastroenterologists see patients in clinic and on hospital rounds on a daily basis, the modern practice of gastroenterology relies heavily on the use of a variety of endoscopes in many contexts. These devices literally revolutionized gastroenterology. Before the development of the modern endoscope, gastroenterologists were limited to using noninvasive testing such as blood tests and physical examinations, radiography in the form of contrast studies, and, later, computed tomography (CT) scans and magnetic resonance imaging (MRI) to assess patients with known or suspected gastrointestinal disease.

Adler DG. *The Little GI Book: An Easily Digestible Guide to Understanding Gastroenterology, Second Edition* (pp 225-272).
© 2020 Taylor & Francis Group.

Endoscopy freed gastroenterologists to perform direct endoscopic examinations of the esophagus, stomach, small intestine, large intestine, pancreas, and bile ducts. Although early endoscopes only had the capacity to perform simple diagnostic maneuvers such as direct visualization of the gastrointestinal tract with the performance of mucosal biopsies, modern endoscopes are fully diagnostic and therapeutic devices that can be used with a tremendous array of endoscopic accessories. Many procedures currently performed via endoscopy could only be performed by surgical approaches in the past. This chapter will review the different endoscopic technologies currently available and will serve as an outline and guide for proper procedure selection in various clinical situations.

THE ENDOSCOPY TEAM

Endoscopy cannot be performed by just one individual. It takes a team working together to perform just about any endoscopic examination. Simple procedures typically require 3 individuals: an endoscopist to physically operate the endoscope; a nurse to sedate the patient and monitor their vital signs including their heart rate, blood pressure, oxygen saturation, and electrocardiogram; and a technician (often a certified medical assistant or another nurse) to set up the equipment, help the endoscopist operate endoscopic accessories, handle biopsy specimens, and perform other tasks. More complicated procedures such as endoscopic retrograde cholangiopancreatography (ERCP) often require multiple assistants given the more complex nature of the procedure being performed and the accessories used.

SEDATION

A full discussion of sedation during endoscopy is beyond the scope of this text, but it is worth noting that different endoscopic procedures require different levels of sedation. Some procedures require no sedation (transnasal upper endoscopy and, in some cases, colonoscopy are performed without any sedation at all), whereas other procedures require general anesthesia with endotracheal intubation performed by an anesthesiologist. Having said that, most procedures are performed using what is referred to as *moderate sedation* (a state in which the patient is relaxed and comfortable and may be sleeping, somewhere between where one might be with no sedation and with general anesthesia) with a combination of sedatives and analgesics. Sedation practices vary from institution to institution and from state to state. There is no gold standard for any particular procedure. The decision of how to sedate a given patient for a particular procedure is often highly individualized.

INFORMED CONSENT

Although extremely safe overall, every endoscopic procedure involves risk, and all endoscopic procedures involve a discussion of the risks and benefits of the procedure with the patient (or a responsible individual if the patient is a minor or too ill to understand) before starting the procedure. A typical informed consent discussion will review the indication for the procedure; a description of what the procedure entails; and the risks, benefits, and alternatives to the procedure. Most institutions will require that the patient or his or her advocate sign a consent form before starting the procedure.

Standard risks of endoscopy include bleeding, allergic/cardiac/respiratory reactions to sedation, bleeding, and perforation (which may warrant surgery). Other procedures carry specific risks beyond the standard ones and will be discussed next.

ESOPHAGOGASTRODUODENOSCOPY

Esophagogastroduodenoscopy (EGD) involves the insertion of an upper endoscope through the patient's mouth to evaluate his or her entire esophagus, entire stomach, and part of the duodenum. Standard EGD typically involves the endoscope being advanced to the level of the second or third portion of the duodenum. The more distal duodenum is typically not evaluated during a standard EGD given the short length of the endoscope.

EGD represents the simplest form of endoscopy and is generally the easiest to learn and the quickest to perform. An experienced endoscopist can perform a complete EGD examination in just a few minutes with a very high degree of diagnostic accuracy.

Standard Upper Endoscope

The standard upper endoscope can be considered the base model from which all other endoscopes are derived. A standard upper endoscope is approximately 1 cm in diameter and has a 4-way tip deflection, a wide field of view, a fiber-optic light source, a camera to generate images, a lens washing feature, and an access channel (often referred to as a *biopsy channel*) through which accessories can be advanced into the patient and fluid can be suctioned into the endoscope. The control head of the endoscope consists of ratchets that control the up/down and left/right movement of the tip of the endoscope, a port for the biopsy channel (covered with a plastic cap), and manually controlled finger valves that regulate the flow of air and water in and out of the endoscope space and also allow the endoscopist to clean the lens if it becomes soiled during a procedure.

Therapeutic Upper Endoscope

So-called *therapeutic upper endoscopes* are available for use in special situations. These devices are identical to standard upper endoscopes with the exception of having a larger cross-sectional diameter and a wider access channel to allow the use of certain therapeutic devices. The wider access channel also allows them to suction fluid more efficiently. Conversely, "ultrathin" endoscopes are available for use in pediatric patients or in patients with strictures that could not be traversed with a standard endoscope. These ultrathin scopes are approximately 5 mm wide and can be inserted transnasally as well. These ultrathin scopes are so small that many patients do not require sedation when they are used to perform an EGD examination.

The upper endoscope itself, like all endoscopes, is coated in a waterproof lining and is a reusable device that must be sterilized between each and every use. Endoscopes are sterilized by a combination of manual washing and a machine-based wash using special chemicals to sterilize the external portion of the endoscope as well as the inside of the biopsy channel.

Diagnostic Upper Endoscopy

Most EGD examinations would be referred to as *diagnostic upper endoscopy*. These examinations are performed in stable patients who need investigation of one or more gastrointestinal complaints. Diagnostic upper endoscopy is also often performed to obtain biopsies of the esophagus, stomach, or small bowel. Some common indications for diagnostic EGD are as follows:

- Evaluation of patients with upper abdominal pain

- Evaluation of patients with known or suspected gastroesophageal reflux disease
- Evaluation of patients with known or suspected peptic ulcer disease
- Evaluation of patients with known or suspected upper gastrointestinal malignancies to obtain biopsies
- Evaluation of patients with dysphagia
- Evaluation of patients with odynophagia (pain with swallowing)
- Evaluation of patients with known or suspected celiac disease and/or chronic diarrhea in order to obtain duodenal biopsies
- Evaluation of patients with weight loss of unclear origin
- Evaluation of patients with anemia of presumed gastrointestinal etiology
- Evaluation of patients with cirrhosis for the presence or absence of esophageal or gastric varices (Figure 8-1)
- Evaluation of the ampulla of Vater in patients with known or suspected ampullary disease (ie, ampullary tumors or cancers)

Therapeutic Upper Endoscopy

Unlike patients undergoing diagnostic upper endoscopy, patients undergoing therapeutic upper endoscopy often have a clinically well-defined problem that needs a therapeutic intervention. Many of these patients are acutely ill, and therapeutic upper endoscopy is often performed on an urgent or emergent, rather than elective, basis. Some indications for therapeutic upper endoscopy are as follows:

- Dilation of esophageal, gastric, or duodenal strictures

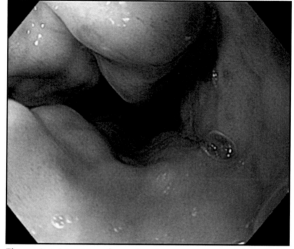

Figure 8-1. Large esophageal varices seen on screening EGD in a patient with cirrhosis.

- Diagnosis and treatment of patients with upper gastrointestinal bleeding
- Placement of esophageal, gastric, or duodenal stents
- Treatment of esophageal or gastric varices via band ligation or sclerotherapy
- Removal of ingested foreign bodies of the esophagus and/or stomach
- Placement of feeding tubes (eg, percutaneous endoscopic gastrostomy [PEG], percutaneous endoscopic jejunostomy)
- Use of thermal therapy to ablate or destroy upper gastrointestinal lesions. (Thermal therapy uses very hot or very cold devices or substances; human tissue dies when exposed to extremely high or low temperatures.) The use of extremely low temperature substances to destroy tissue is known as *cryotherapy*.

In all fairness, I should point out that these lists are somewhat artificial. It is often difficult to know before you put the endoscope into the patient's mouth exactly what you are going to find and what sort of procedure you will need to be doing (ie, the patient complaining of abdominal pain may be referred for diagnostic EGD only to discover that the patient has a large bezoar in his or her stomach). A bezoar is a nondigestible foreign body (usually made of ingested vegetable matter, hair, or other substances). Bezoars are typically removed endoscopically, but the removal of such a structure essentially constitutes a therapeutic upper endoscopy. Similarly, a patient may complain of dysphasia that prompts an EGD to be performed. The EGD might result in the discovery of a high-grade esophageal stricture that the endoscopist dilates during the same procedure—again illustrating how a diagnostic procedure can quickly become a therapeutic procedure. Conversely, sometimes a procedure intended to be therapeutic will be only diagnostic in nature (ie, a patient will describe symptoms of upper gastrointestinal bleeding that warrant a therapeutic procedure only to discover that the patient has a normal examination endoscopically and that no therapeutic maneuvers are required). Most endoscopists are trained in both diagnostic and therapeutic endoscopy and should be able to handle most (if not all) situations that could potentially arise during the course of an EGD.

It is also worth mentioning that most EGDs involve a maneuver known as *retroflexion*. This means that the endoscope is bent back on itself (like an umbrella handle) so that the most proximal portion of the stomach (the gastric cardia) can be directly visualized.

COLONOSCOPY

Colonoscopy is an endoscopic examination of the colon. While often the punch line to a stand-up comedian's joke or a source of humor on a sitcom, colonoscopy is actually serious business. Colonoscopy is a complex procedure that requires significant skill on the part of the endoscopist. Colonoscopy also takes quite a lot of time to master from a technical point of view, and physicians who perform colonoscopy will often accrue hundreds of supervised procedures under their belts before they complete their training. It is not uncommon for an experienced gastroenterologist to perform many thousands of colonoscopy procedures over the course of his or her career (it is actually not too difficult to reach a personal experience of performing over 20,000 colonoscopies during one's career as a gastroenterologist!). Most importantly, colonoscopy has been definitively shown to reduce deaths from colorectal cancer.

Colonoscopy is most commonly performed with a standard adult colonoscope. This is a wider and stiffer instrument than used for an EGD, but it operates in a very similar manner to an upper endoscope. The colonoscope also has a large working channel to allow passage of accessories for various endoscopic maneuvers. Although an EGD involves passage through a relatively straight segment of the gastrointestinal tract, the colonoscopist must drive the colonoscope through the twists and turns of the large bowel, which can often be severe. The colonoscope is prone to forming loops, which can retard advancement and are often very uncomfortable for the patient undergoing the procedure. A loop can sometimes result in the development of what is known as *paradoxical motion*. Paradoxical motion occurs when a large loop has formed in the endoscope, and further advancement of the instrument results in a backwards motion of the tip of the endoscope. Colonoscopy often involves a constant effort to keep the colonoscope straight so that the endoscopist can achieve one-to-one motion (1 cm of colonoscope advancement results in moving 1 cm further into the colon). Keeping the colonoscope straight generally involves reducing the scope (also known as *pulling back*) to prevent the formation of loops or to get rid of them if they occur. Thus, physicians often feel as if they are pulling their way through the colon rather than pushing their way through.

A typical colonoscopy involves complete endoscopic examination of the entire colon from the anus to the cecum (the most proximal part of the colon). It is not uncommon for a colonoscopy to involve direct visualization and intubation of the terminal ileum (the most distal portion of the small bowel that empties into the cecum via the ileocecal valve) as well. A colonoscopy usually involves a retroflexion in the rectum to visualize the most distal portion of the colon, just as an EGD examination usually includes a retroflexion to view the most proximal portion of the stomach.

Colonoscopy also involves a digital rectal examination. A digital rectal examination involves the endoscopist inserting his or her index finger into the rectum through the anus to assess sphincter tone and for the presence of any palpable masses or lesions in the distal rectum.

Types

Screening Colonoscopy

A screening colonoscopy is performed on an asymptomatic individual to evaluate him or her for the presence of polyps (the precursor lesions to colorectal cancer). Any polyps seen during a screening colonoscopy are generally removed during the procedure unless they are felt to be too large to safely removed with an endoscope. Most guidelines suggest that average-risk patients should begin screening at age 50. If the colonoscopy is performed and the patient has no disease or polyps, the examination is repeated at intervals based on factors such as the patient's family history, quality of the examination, etc. A typical interval between negative screening colonoscopies is 5 to 10 years.

Surveillance Colonoscopy

Surveillance colonoscopy involves the endoscopic evaluation of the colon in a patient who has a prior history of colonic disease. The most common indication for a surveillance colonoscopy is to reevaluate someone who had adenomatous polyps on a prior colonoscopy (ie, those who developed polyps in the past are more likely to develop them in the future, and these patients are typically examined at more frequent intervals). Some common indications for surveillance colonoscopy are as follows:

- Personal history of colonic polyps
- Personal history of colon or rectal cancer after removal
- Personal history of inflammatory bowel disease (ulcerative colitis or Crohn's disease, the presence of which can increase your risk of colorectal cancer)

Diagnostic Colonoscopy

Diagnostic colonoscopy is performed when a patient develops symptoms that are suggestive of primary colorectal disease or in those patients in whom the terminal ileum is thought to be the source of disease (eg, the terminal ileum is a frequent site of inflammation in patients with Crohn's disease). Some common indications for diagnostic colonoscopy are as follows:

- Lower abdominal pain
- Investigation of past episodes of the passage of bright red blood per rectum, also known as *hematochezia* (Figure 8-2)

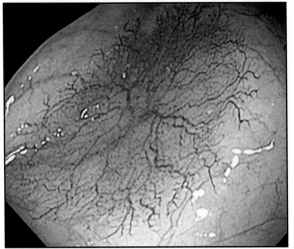

Figure 8-2. Rectal arteriovenous malformation seen in a patient with hematochezia. Arteriovenous malformations like this one often periodically bleed spontaneously. These can be ablated via thermal therapy during colonoscopy.

- Known or suspected ulcerative colitis
- Known or suspected Crohn's disease
- Known or suspected diverticular disease (also known as *diverticulosis* [but generally not *acute diverticulitis*])
- Anemia of presumed gastrointestinal origin
- Positive fecal occult blood test
- Chronic diarrhea
- Weight loss of unclear etiology
- Chronic constipation
- Fecal incontinence

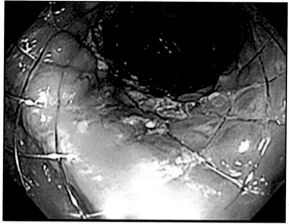

Figure 8-3. A colonic stent placed to relieve obstruction from a colon cancer.

Therapeutic Colonoscopy

Therapeutic colonoscopy, as the name suggests, involves performing a colonoscopy with the intent of doing a specific therapeutic maneuver or maneuvers in a patient with a previously diagnosed problem. Many of these procedures are performed in acutely ill patients who are already hospitalized. Some common indications for therapeutic colonoscopy are as follows:

- The treatment of active lower gastrointestinal bleeding (usually hematochezia, but this can also be performed for patients with melena who have had a negative EGD)
- Decompression of patients with an obstructing colon cancer via the placement of a stent or a colon decompression tube (Figure 8-3)
- Decompression of patients with functional colonic obstruction (known as *Ogilvie's syndrome*) via placement of a decompression tube

- Decompression of patients with a sigmoid or cecal volvulus (where the bowel twists onto itself like the ends of a sausage casing); colonoscopy can often succeed in untwisting the bowel in this setting, or a decompression tube can be used as well

- Endoscopic removal of large polyps using specialized polypectomy techniques

- Use of thermal therapy to ablate or destroy lower gastrointestinal lesions

Polypectomy

A full discussion of polypectomy is beyond the range of this book (there are entire books devoted to the subject), but it is worth mentioning that polypectomy is, by far, the most common therapeutic technique applied during colonoscopy. Polypectomy refers to the endoscopic removal of colorectal polyps. These polyps are usually adenomatous (glandular) polyps—the most common precursor lesions to colorectal cancers. Once a polyp is completely removed from a patient, it cannot develop further into a colorectal cancer.

Polypectomy techniques and tools abound. We can discuss some of the more common ones here. Simple "cold" forceps (that do not use electrocautery during polypectomy) are used to simply grab and pull small polyps off of the bowel wall. Snares, which resemble a cowboy's lasso, can be placed over a polyp and used to cut the polyp off intact or in several pieces. "Hot" and cold snares are available and are in widespread use. Other techniques involve injecting liquids into the submucosal space to lift an overlying polyp and to create a cushion of fluid underneath the polyp. This submucosal fluid cushion allows the polyp to be removed more safely because the underlying muscle and adventitia of the colon are separated from the polyp itself during the polypectomy; this reduces the risk of a perforation. In the past and even today, the most common agent used to create a submucosal fluid cushion was simple saline, but now specialized submucosal lifting agents are commercially available that make better, bigger cushions that last longer (saline gets reabsorbed by the body quickly, limiting the time for the polypectomy). These new specialized lifting agents really do work much better than saline but are significantly more expensive than saline. As such, saline is still widely used, but the newer lifting agents are starting to be more widely adopted. Endoscopic clips can be used to treat postpolypectomy bleeding and to close the lining of the colon after a large polyp has been removed. These clips can also be used to seal a perforation in some cases.

Tools to Enhance Polyp Detection

Recent years have seen a rise in the development and availability of specialized tools and techniques to assist during colonoscopy, mostly to improve polyp detection rates overall. These tools all appear to be safe and to work but do increase the cost of colonoscopy because an extra device is usually required. Some of the most common tools and techniques to enhance polyp detection are shown in Figure 8-4 and include the following:

- **Retroflexion in the right colon:** This does not add cost but allows the endoscopist to the see the right colon, an area of particular concern, from a different vantage point.

- **Two trips through the right colon:** Evaluating the right colon twice also does not add cost, just time, but may help to identify polyps missed on a single evaluation of the right colon.

- **Fixation of a clear cap to the colonoscope tip:** A simple clear cap can be used to help flatten out colonic folds. This sounds simple, but it is actually quite effective.

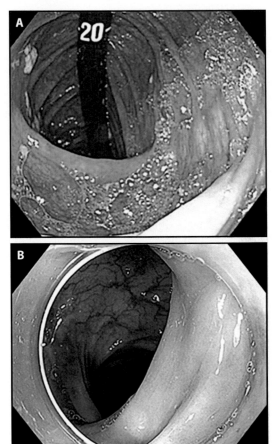

Figure 8-4. Some devices and maneuvers to increase polyp detection during colonoscopy. (A) Retroflexion in the right colon. (B) A clear cap affixed to the end of the colonoscope to flatten folds. (*continued*)

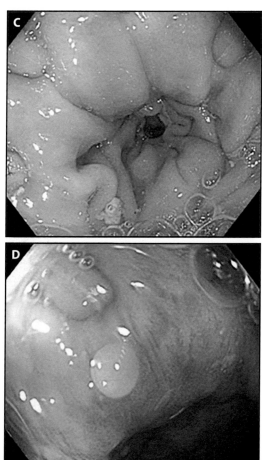

Figure 8-4 (continued). (C) A cap with finger-like projections affixed to the end of the colonoscope to flatten folds. (D) The same cap as used in C showing how the finger-like projections helped identify a small polyp that might otherwise have been missed.

- **Fixation of a cap with rings or finger-like projections:** Modified caps have appendages that "reach out" and can further help to flatten out colonic folds to help identify polyps that might be otherwise missed.

- **Miniature endoscopes that look in the opposite direction of the colonoscope:** These devices allow the endoscopist to see both forward- and backward-looking views simultaneously to help identify more polyps for removal.

CAPSULE ENDOSCOPY

Capsule endoscopy represents one of the newest additions to the endoscopist's tool bag. As the name suggests, capsule endoscopy uses miniature capsule-shaped endoscopes to visualize the bowel. These capsule endoscopes are generally about 1 inch long and a little less than half an inch wide. Unlike the other endoscopes that we will discuss in this chapter, capsule endoscopes are not directly operated by a physician. Once activated, the patient swallows the capsule, which contains its own power and light source, camera, and lens. The capsule then takes pictures at a predetermined rate as it passes through the esophagus, stomach, small bowel, and colon. A typical capsule endoscope will take many thousands of pictures on its journey through the patient's digestive tract. Interestingly, the capsule itself does not store these pictures; it transmits them through a series of antenna leads the patient wears around his or her abdomen to a recorder unit that the patient wears on his or her belt.

Capsule endoscopes are disposable items; these are the only nonreusable endoscopes in all of gastrointestinal endoscopy, although that may change in the future. Once the battery power in the capsule is depleted, it simply stops taking pictures and ceases transmitting them to the recorder unit. In most cases, the patient simply passes the capsule along with a bowel movement at a later time. Most patients do not even know that they have passed the capsule when it actually happens. Depending on the patient, it can take hours or days for the capsule to transit the bowel. In rare cases, the capsule can become trapped in the patient's intestine. This typically occurs in patients with strictures or inflammatory bowel disease, such as Crohn's disease. Trapped capsule endoscopes sometimes need to be retrieved either endoscopically or surgically, although many times the trapped capsule will eventually pass through an obstructing stricture on its own without outside intervention.

We have already discussed how upper endoscopes and colonoscopes do an excellent job of visualizing the esophagus, stomach, proximal small bowel, terminal ileum, and the entire colon and rectum. Capsule endoscopes, although useful for a variety of purposes, are primarily used to investigate the small bowel that lies between what is reachable by standard upper endoscopy and a colonoscopy. The small bowel is quite long and can exceed a length of 20 feet in an average adult. The small bowel is tortuous in course, thin walled, and not fixed in the abdomen like some other portions of the gastrointestinal tract (ie, the duodenum). Historically, patients with suspected small bowel disease were investigated by radiographs, such as a small bowel follow-through (where the patient drank some form of contrast and X-rays were obtained as it passed through the patient's intestines to generate images). Capsule endoscopy revolutionized small bowel imaging; for the first time, physicians were able to obtain high-resolution, mucosal-based, color images of the entire small bowel in a relatively noninvasive manner. Patients undergoing capsule endoscopy require no sedation, and they do not even have to stay in the hospital during the procedure; they are free to go about their business, including driving and going to work. As the capsule transits the small bowel, it transmits the images it obtains to the recorder unit as described previously. The following day, the patient simply returns the antenna leads and the recording device to the hospital and waits for results.

Once the physician receives the recording device and the antenna leads back from the patient, the leads themselves are recycled for use in another patient and the recording device, which contains the images obtained during the capsule endoscopy examination, is linked to a computer into which the images are downloaded. Using software provided by the manufacturer of the capsule endoscope, the thousands of images obtained during the capsule endoscopy procedure are assembled into a video that can be watched on a computer.

When viewing capsule endoscopy video on a monitor, the physician generally watches the video from start to finish, looking for signs of pathology. The overwhelming majority of capsule endoscopy procedures are performed to investigate the small bowel. Special capsule endoscopes that specifically look at either the esophagus or the colon exist, but these are used much less frequently than the small bowel capsules. Thus, almost all capsule endoscopes these days result in a video of the small intestine that is closely studied to look for pathology. I have reviewed hundreds of capsule endoscopy videos, and well over 90% of them were done to investigate the small bowel.

The most common indication for capsule endoscopy has been and remains the investigation of occult or obscure gastrointestinal bleeding thought to arise from the small bowel. Another common indication for capsule endoscopy is to look for signs of Crohn's disease in a patient suspected to have inflammatory bowel disease in whom other forms of endoscopy have been unrevealing.

The capsule endoscope, using data from the antenna leads, also generates a crude 2-dimensional map of the patient's abdomen. Combining this map with the transit time of the capsule as it passes to the small bowel often gives the physician a rough idea of where to look in the patient's intestines when following up with an actual endoscope for any abnormality seen during a capsule study.

It is very common to find ulcers, angioectasias (abnormal mucosal blood vessels that can bleed), polyps, and signs of Crohn's disease when viewing a capsule endoscopy examination of the small bowel. Less commonly, tumors and/or strictures are encountered. Unfortunately, sometimes the examination is unrevealing, even when the patient is known to have active small bowel disease. The most typical example of this is a patient with known small bowel bleeding in whom a capsule study is unremarkable. Sometimes patients have to have multiple capsule studies before a bleeding source can be identified; this can be intensely frustrating for both the patient and the physician.

Sometimes a lesion is found that warrants surgery (eg, a tumor). Other times a source of bleeding such as an ulcer or an angioectasia is identified. Capsule endoscopes have no therapeutic capability. To perform therapeutic maneuvers in the small bowel, one needs to perform an enteroscopy, usually with the application of some form of thermal therapy to destroy the lesion in question or maneuvers to biopsy or remove the lesion.

In the past, there was only one type of capsule endoscope on the market, and now there are many. Some capsule endoscopes are meant to image the small bowel, and some are made to just visualize the colon. Some have one camera, and some have two cameras. Some can even transmit their images in real time so an observer can watch what the camera is seeing as it moves through the bowel.

ENTEROSCOPY

Enteroscopy refers to the use of special endoscopes to directly investigate the small bowel. We have already established that upper endoscopy and colonoscopy both investigate the small bowel to only a limited extent. Upper endoscopy typically involves investigation of the proximal portion of the duodenum. Colonoscopy often (but not always!) involves examination of the terminal ileum (the very last portion of the small bowel). At best, performing standard upper and lower endoscopy will allow the endoscopist to evaluate only this very small portion of the small bowel. As mentioned earlier, many adults will have up to 20 feet of small intestine. Enteroscopy refers to procedures that are specifically designed to go deep into the small bowel (either from above or below) for dedicated small bowel investigations and therapy.

Most enteroscopy procedures are performed for a relatively limited number of indications. The most common indication for an enteroscopy procedure is to investigate bleeding presumed to be of small bowel origin. Many, if not most, patients undergo capsule endoscopy before undergoing enteroscopy, and many enteroscopy procedures are performed based on the positive findings of a capsule endoscopy. Other common indications for enteroscopy include the investigation of patients with known or suspected Crohn's disease or patients with known or suspected small bowel tumors.

A variety of specialty scopes can be used to investigate the small bowel, including the following:

Colonoscope

A colonoscope can be inserted by mouth (per os) to reach the small bowel from above. The use of a colonoscope from above probably represents the most commonly performed procedure to investigate the small bowel. Advantages of using a colonoscope in this manner include the widespread availability of the device, ease of use, and an endoscope length and working channel diameter that will accommodate essentially any endoscopic accessory.

Push Enteroscope

A push enteroscope is a special endoscope with a very long length. Most push enteroscopes are either 240 or 250 cm long. Compare this with the 140-cm length for a standard colonoscope, and you can see that this is a device designed for deep evaluation of the small bowel. These devices can be inserted by mouth or through the patient's anus for investigation of the small bowel from below (if inserted from below, the endoscopist first has to traverse the entire colon and then begin a retrograde examination of the small bowel). When inserted from above, a push enteroscope can often reach distances of 80 cm beyond the pylorus and sometimes further. Conversely, a colonoscope can typically only investigate 10 to 20 cm of the terminal ileum before the endoscopist literally runs out of scope. Using a push enteroscope from below, one can often investigate 50 to 100 cm of the distal small bowel. It is very difficult to investigate the entire small bowel with a push enteroscope, and you can see that even paired investigations from above and below in the same patient will likely leave some small bowel in the middle unvisualized. Still, push enteroscopes are valuable devices that are often quite successful, allowing a physician to reach sites of small bowel pathology and perform some sort of diagnostic and/or therapeutic maneuver.

Because of their great length, push enteroscopes require special endoscopic accessories. Standard accessories are simply not long enough to use with these devices. There are a limited number of accessories for push enteroscopes, including biopsy forceps, special catheters to deliver thermal energy to destroy tissue, and snares to perform polypectomy. Push enteroscopes are often limited in their ability to reach deep areas of the small bowel by the formation of loops. When inserted from above, it is very common for the enteroscope to loop in the stomach. This loop reduces the depth to which the enteroscope can reach, causes pain and discomfort to the patient, and may result in paradoxical motion as is seen during colonoscopy. If the enteroscope is inserted from below, loops can form in the colon just as they do during colonoscopy. When performing push enteroscopy, one of the main jobs of the endoscopist is to always be on the lookout for the formation of loops and reduce these appropriately as they occur. This may require external pressure from an assistant.

Balloon Enteroscopy

Balloon enteroscopy refers to a branch of gastrointestinal endoscopy that uses special enteroscopes that can reach into the distal small bowel and can potentially investigate a patient's entire small bowel (Figure 8-5). Double-balloon enteroscopy refers to the use of a special enteroscope that comes with a long, flexible overtube. In double-balloon enteroscopy, both the enteroscope and the overtube have balloons (that can be inflated or deflated) affixed to the tips. The overtube helps minimize loop formation (given its stiffness). The balloons on the tip of the overtube and the endoscope help to fix the position of these devices during a maneuver known as a *reduction*. A reduction involves withdrawing the overtube and the enteroscope together to both reduce any loops that may have formed and to allow pleating of the bowel around the enteroscope. Pleating of the bowel refers to an accordion-like compression of the bowel around the endoscope, which produces a functional shortening of the bowel and allows for deep advancement into the small bowel.

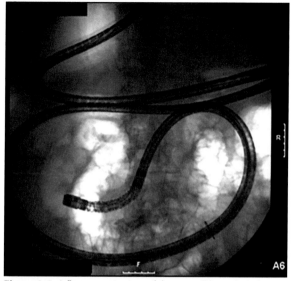

Figure 8-5. A fluoroscopic view of deep small bowel intubation using a double-balloon endoscope.

Single-balloon enteroscopy refers to a competing system that is very similar to double-balloon enteroscopy. Both of these systems use special enteroscopes as well as overtubes, but single-balloon enteroscopy (as the name suggests) only involves a single balloon, which is affixed to the end of the overtube.

Balloon enteroscopy procedures can be very time consuming. It is not uncommon for a balloon enteroscopy procedure to require 2 or more hours to perform. Experienced balloon enteroscopists can perform a deep examination of the small bowel in 1 hour, but it takes time to develop this skill. There are many reports of physicians using balloon enteroscopy to examine the entire small bowel in one procedure, although most balloon enteroscopy procedures are not quite this successful, and most endoscopists are not quite that patient!

Balloon enteroscopy is also physically demanding on the endoscopist because the procedure requires multiple steps performed in a specific order to be repeated many times (ie, steps such as advancement of the enteroscope, inflation and deflation of the balloons at the appropriate times, withdrawal of the enteroscope and the overtube at the appropriate time in the appropriate manner need to be performed correctly over and over again over a long period of time). This can leave the endoscopist and his or her assistants physically drained and worn out after the procedure, especially if the anatomy is challenging!

ENDOSCOPIC RETROGRADE CHOLANGIOPANCREATOGRAPHY

ERCP has been and remains the most complex and challenging procedure in all of gastrointestinal endoscopy. ERCP is also the most misunderstood procedure in the sense that physicians who do not perform ERCP will often have misperceptions about what ERCP is, who it is for, who should do it, and what it can and cannot accomplish.

The term *ERCP* refers to a set of endoscopic interventions on the pancreas and/or bile ducts to both diagnose and treat pancreaticobiliary disease. ERCP uses a special endoscope referred to as a *duodenoscope* combined with simultaneous fluoroscopy. The duodenoscope is used to insert devices into the bile and/or pancreatic ducts, and the fluoroscope is used to visualize those devices and injected contrast dye once they are within the liver and the pancreas themselves (which are generally not directly visualized).

The duodenoscope is unique in that its optical lens is positioned 90 degrees off-axis; specifically, the duodenoscope is a side-viewing instrument. The duodenoscope is designed this way because ERCP is almost always performed with the tip of the duodenoscope in the second portion of the duodenum facing the ampulla of Vater (the structure at which the distal common bile duct and the pancreatic duct terminate and where bile and pancreatic juice are released into the small bowel to help break down food in the small intestine). Because the duodenoscope is a side-viewing instrument, when using it, you cannot go where you are looking, and you cannot look where you are going. Confused? Tomorrow, when you drive to work or school, imagine if you had to paint your windshield over with black paint and make your daily drive with only the view out of the passenger's front window to guide you. Impossible? No. Difficult? Yes. The trick is that you could probably do it if you had driven the route enough times already and had a good sense of what was likely to be around you at any given time.

The duodenoscope also has, in addition to 4-way tip deflection control ratchets, a special control referred to as an *elevator*. The elevator is a small lever built into the tip of the duodenoscope that allows the operator to lift and lower endoscopic accessories that have been passed through the working channel. The elevator, as simple as it may sound, gives the duodenoscope an additional degree of freedom and is of critical value in performing ERCP maneuvers.

The side-viewing nature of the duodenoscope also changes the nature of the control ratchets. The up/down ratchet now deflects the tip of the endoscope either closer to or farther from the duodenal wall, and the right/left ratchet now rotates the endoscopic image clockwise or counterclockwise.

Most training programs reserve ERCP training to senior fellows (or special advanced fellows) who have already demonstrated proficiency with standard endoscopes over hundreds or thousands of procedures. Even experienced endoscopists can find their first encounter with a duodenoscope to be a humbling experience as they try to drive an endoscope that looks familiar but in an alien manner in their hands.

Modern imaging studies such as MRI and CT scanning have largely rendered so-called *diagnostic ERCP* a thing of the past. Almost (but not quite) all ERCP procedures currently performed are therapeutic in nature. This means that a specific problem or group of problems has been identified in a given patient, and the ERCP is performed with very specific goals. This is in contrast to much of the rest of endoscopy, where diagnostic procedures are commonly performed. The reason for the dearth of diagnostic ERCP procedures is that an ERCP carries, on average, more inherent risk than any other endoscopic procedure. As such, there is a strong emphasis placed on proper patient selection in ERCP to avoid unnecessary procedures in an attempt to minimize complications.

In addition to all of the standard risks of endoscopy, ERCP carries a significant risk of causing pancreatitis (specifically referred to as *post-ERCP pancreatitis* [PEP]). An average-risk ERCP carries about a 4% to 7% risk of pancreatitis, but some specific ERCP procedures can have a much higher risk of causing PEP. PEP can be mild, moderate, or severe in nature and in rare instances can be fatal. Most patients who develop PEP will require hospitalization for several days while they recover. Experienced ERCP practitioners can have very low rates of PEP, but as of this writing, there is no way to completely eliminate the risk of PEP. At many institutions, patients undergoing ERCP also receive a dose of the nonsteroidal anti-inflammatory drug indomethacin before each ERCP because this agent has been shown to reduce the risk of PEP.

ERCP also uses very specialized tools and accessories given the nature of the work involved. Most ERCP procedures involve the passage of accessories through the endoscope and through the ampulla of Vater into the bile ducts and/or the pancreatic ducts where they then perform their primary function.

Accessories

ERCP requires specific accessories not used in other endoscopic procedures. Some common ERCP accessories include the following:

- **Guidewires:** ERCP relies heavily on guidewires to secure access to the desired ductal system (biliary or pancreatic) and over which different endoscopic accessories can be advanced or withdrawn. Guidewires are often advanced into very specific locations in the ducts in order to allow accessories to reach these specific locations repeatedly and easily. Guidewires range from 0.018 to 0.035 inches (ie, 18/1000 of an inch to 35/1000 of an inch, respectively).

- **Cannulas:** These are straight catheters used to access the bile and pancreatic ducts. They can inject and aspirate dye or other fluids into the ducts. Injected dye is visible only via fluoroscopy. Guidewires can pass through cannulas.

- **Sphincterotomes:** Sphincterotomes are specialized catheters that, in addition to allowing for the injection of dye and the passage of guidewires, contain a special cutting wire that allows endoscopists to perform a sphincterotomy. The cutting wire, when tensed via a hand control, bows the tip of the sphincterotome. This bowing motion is often helpful during the selective cannulation of the bile or pancreatic ducts. The term *sphincterotomy* generally refers to the use of this cutting wire to transmit energy (in the form of electrocautery) to the tissue of the sphincter of Oddi. The sphincter of Oddi refers to the muscular sphincter complex that regulates the flow of bile and pancreatic juice into the small bowel. Many ERCP procedures depend on the ability to ablate these muscular sphincters.

- **Balloons:** ERCP balloons come in 2 varieties know as *occlusion balloons* and *dilating balloons.* Occlusion balloons are inflated to match the diameter of the surrounding duct. Once inflated, these balloons can be used to sweep the duct of any sludge, stones, or debris or can be used to perform an occlusion study wherein injected dye is prevented from flowing above or below the balloon. Occlusion studies are often very helpful for delineating pancreaticobiliary anatomy because the balloon holds the dye in the desired duct for as long as desired so that adequate visualization of these structures is obtained. Dilating balloons, as their name suggests, are used to dilate strictures that occur in the ducts.

- **Baskets:** Baskets are ERCP devices that are most commonly used to retrieve stones from the ducts. Baskets come in many shapes and designs. Some baskets are simple graspers, whereas others are capable of crushing stones and are referred to as *lithotripters* (Figure 8-6).

- **Stents:** Stents are devices that are generally used to hold a blocked or strictured duct open. Stents can be made of plastic or a flexible metal mesh. Metal stents can be made of meshes that consist of bare wire, partially covered wire, or fully covered wire. Plastic stents are generally considered

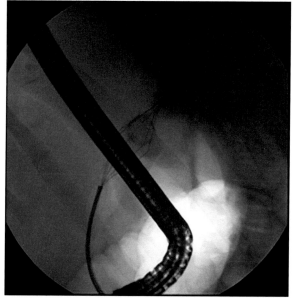

Figure 8-6. A fluoroscopic view of a large stone in a biliary stone basket during ERCP.

temporary devices. Metal stents can be placed on a temporary or permanent basis (Figure 8-7).

- **Brushes:** ERCP brushes are wire brushes contained within a catheter. When advanced over a guidewire to a desired location (usually a stricture), the brush can be scraped across the stricture in an attempt to capture cells, which can be evaluated by a specialized pathologist known as a *cytologist* to look for the presence of cancer.
- **Cholangioscopes and pancreatoscopes:** These devices are miniaturized endoscopes that can be advanced into the bile ducts and pancreatic

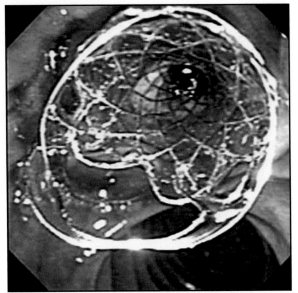

Figure 8-7. An endoscopic view of a biliary self-expanding metal stent after deployment across the ampulla in a patient with a bile duct stricture due to pancreatic cancer.

ducts for direct visualization of these structures (Figure 8-8). In the past, these devices were fiber-optic cameras, but modern versions are digital, which produce much sharper and brighter images. Cholangioscopes and pancreatoscopes can be used to locate tumors, take tissue samples, and break up stones. In the past, these devices were rarely purchased and cumbersome to use. Modern cholangioscopes and pancreatoscopes have much better optical quality and are much easier for the physician to operate during ERCP. These devices add to the invasiveness of ERCP, but if used properly, they do not add to the overall risk of the procedure.

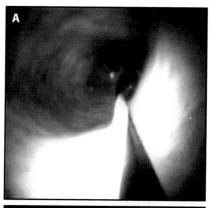

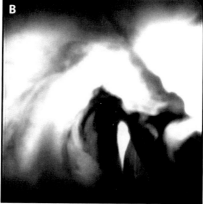

Figure 8-8. Cholangioscopy and pancreatoscopy. (A) A digital cholangioscopic image of a normal, healthy bile duct. Note the uniform walls and widely patent duct. A guidewire is visible as well. For scale, the guidewire is 0.025 inches wide. (B) A digital cholangioscopic image of a bile duct cancer (cholangiocarcinoma). Note the narrow duct with irregular walls. (*continued*)

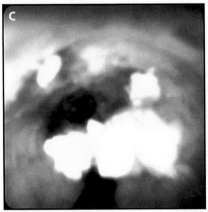

Figure 8-8 (continued). (C) A digital pancreatoscopic image of white pancreatic duct stones in a patient with chronic pancreatitis. The stones were subsequently removed.

Indications

Some common indications for ERCP include the following:

- **Known or suspected bile duct stones (usually causing biliary obstruction and jaundice):** Stones are removed via a combination of biliary sphincterotomy and stone extraction, usually via balloons and baskets (Figure 8-9).
- **Known or suspected bile duct strictures (usually causing biliary obstruction and jaundice):** These strictures can be from cancer, inflammation, or a bile duct injury. Bile duct injuries most commonly occur as a complication of surgery, such as a cholecystectomy.
- **Known or suspected bile leaks:** Bile leaks are common after cholecystectomy and can occur

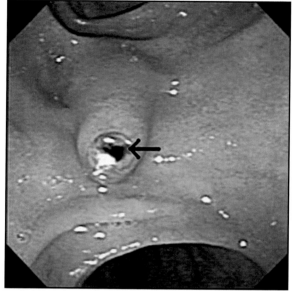

Figure 8-9. An impacted stone (arrow) visible at the ampulla seen during ERCP in a patient with jaundice.

anywhere in the biliary tree but most often occur at the site of the cystic duct remnant (where the gallbladder was separated from the biliary tree). Bile leaks can also occur after liver transplantation or liver resections. Bile leaks allow bile to escape the biliary tree and enter the abdomen, where it can cause pain, inflammation, and infection. ERCP is used to treat bile leaks by using biliary sphincterotomy and/or biliary stents to redirect the flow of bile down to the duodenum where it belongs. As bile stops flowing out of the leak, the leak will heal slowly over the course of several weeks. At that time, stents can be removed because they are no longer needed.

- **Cholangitis:** Cholangitis refers to an infected bile duct. Cholangitis is often a medical emergency and is usually treated by aggressive fluid and antibiotic administration as well as ERCP to drain the bile duct and, thus, drain the infection. Cholangitis can occur in the setting of biliary obstruction (from a clogged stent or an impacted bile duct stone) but can sometimes occur without systemic obstruction (from an infected stent or other foreign body in the bile ducts) or in the context of some specific diseases such as primary sclerosing cholangitis.

- **Chronic pancreatitis:** Some patients with chronic pancreatitis benefit from ERCP, often to remove pancreatic duct stones, dilate strictures, or place pancreatic duct stents. ERCP for chronic pancreatitis is usually only performed by expert endoscopists.

- **Acute pancreatitis:** ERCP in the setting of acute pancreatitis (usually performed to relieve concomitant biliary obstruction) has been and remains controversial and is often performed based on local experience and on a case-by-case basis. Some fear that performing ERCP in a patient with existing pancreatitis might worsen his or her overall situation, whereas others suggest it may speed the patient's recovery.

ENDOSCOPIC ULTRASOUND

Endoscopic ultrasound (EUS) refers to a set of procedures that use echoendoscopes; these are specialized endoscopes that contain not just a light and a camera but an ultrasound transducer as well. EUS allows the endoscopist to perform an ultrasound from the inside of the body (as opposed to transabdominal ultrasound, which is performed through the abdominal wall from the outside of the body).

EUS allows us to see a variety of organs and structures we would not be otherwise able to see with standard "white light" endoscopes. First, EUS allows us to see the individual wall layers that make up the luminal gastro-intestinal tract. This is critical for staging tumors of the esophagus, stomach, and rectum because the staging of these tumors is highly dependent on the deepest wall layer involved with the tumor, and the tumor's stage determines its treatment regimen. Regular endoscopes can only see the mucosal side of these organs, but EUS endoscopes can see all the way through the entire bowel wall. These devices can also look for and biopsy lymph nodes near tumors that are also completely invisible with regular endoscopes. Of critical importance, EUS allows us to see the pancreas, bile ducts, and other extraluminal organs with great clarity. The pancreas has historically been very difficult to clearly visualize (let alone biopsy), and these difficulties have largely been solved by the use of EUS.

Although EUS has a variety of uses, it is most commonly used to diagnose and stage patients with gastro-intestinal cancer. In a single EUS procedure, a tumor can be identified, biopsied, and the extent of disease definitively assessed (staged). EUS is especially helpful in patients with pancreatic cancer because the staging of these patients depends heavily on the relationship of the primary tumor to several key peripancreatic blood vessels, all of which can be identified during EUS. It is worth noting that EUS is often combined with other procedures to save time. For example, in my practice, I often perform EUS and ERCP in one setting for patients with pancreatic cancer in order to perform a needle biopsy of the mass and to relieve obstructive jaundice with a stent (be it metal or plastic). Similarly, I will often perform EUS and

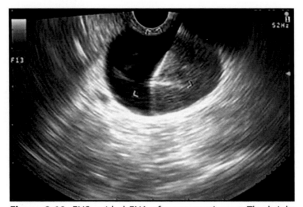

Figure 8-10. EUS-guided FNA of a pancreatic cyst. The bright straight line is the needle itself penetrating the surrounding cyst.

esophageal stenting in patients with esophageal cancer to allow for tumor staging and stenting (to treat dysphagia) all in one procedure.

In many instances, EUS imaging is superior to that of CT scans or MRI in terms of diagnostic accuracy and overall image resolution. Using special EUS scopes, endoscopists can also perform a variety of diagnostic and therapeutic maneuvers. The most common EUS maneuver is to perform a biopsy via a fine-needle aspiration (FNA), usually of a pancreatic mass, pancreatic cyst, or an extraintestinal lymph node (Figure 8-10). These FNAs allow us to easily obtain tissue from organs and structures we would otherwise have great difficulty reaching.

EUS can also perform a variety of therapeutic maneuvers using these same FNA needle devices in an off-label manner. FNA needles can be used to inject a variety of agents for varying purposes into structures outside the luminal gastrointestinal tract that would otherwise be very hard to reach. The best example of this technology is the use of FNA needles to inject anesthetics or alcohol

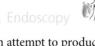

into the celiac nerve in an attempt to produce temporary or permanent pain relief in patients with chronic pancreatitis or pancreatic cancer, respectively. EUS can also be used to drain pancreatic cysts and access the bile ducts or pancreatic ducts in patients in whom ERCP has been unsuccessful or in whom EUS is not technically possible due to anatomic constraints, although these indications are less commonly encountered.

Some common indications for EUS include the following:

- Evaluation, staging, and biopsy of patients with known or suspected esophageal cancer
- Evaluation, staging, and biopsy of patients with known or suspected gastric cancer or gastric lymphoma
- Evaluation, staging, and biopsy of patients with known or suspected pancreatic cancer
- Evaluation, staging, and biopsy of patients with known or suspected rectal cancer
- Evaluation and biopsy of mediastinal lymph nodes or masses
- Evaluation and drainage of pancreatic cystic neoplasms by FNA
- Treatment of abdominal pain in patients with chronic pancreatitis by celiac block
- Treatment of abdominal pain in patients with pancreatic cancer by celiac neurolysis
- Evaluation of patients with abdominal pain for the presence or absence of chronic pancreatitis
- Evaluation and biopsy in patients with submucosal tumors of the esophagus, stomach, or rectum
- Placement of lumen-apposing metal stents (LAMSs) for transluminal procedures (discussed later)
- Evaluation and treatment of patients with bleeding gastric varices via EUS-guided glue or coil injection

FEEDING TUBES

Gastroenterologists are often asked to insert feeding tubes in patients who cannot otherwise eat and/ or swallow normally. This is common in patients who have obstructing lesions in their esophagus who cannot swallow, patients who have head and neck cancers (who also cannot swallow), patients who have had a stroke and cannot swallow safely due to a high risk of aspiration, patients with severe pancreatitis who need to be fed directly into their jejunum (thus bypassing the stomach and small bowel in an attempt to allow the pancreas to avoid stimulation), and in many other situations.

Feeding tubes come in several varieties. Most gastroenterologists are familiar with and can insert most, if not all, of these tubes. These tubes can also be placed by radiologists and surgeons.

- Nasogastric tubes are inserted through the nose and pass into the stomach. These are usually placed in patients with an upper gastrointestinal obstruction who need a short-term feeding tube.

- Nasoenteric tubes are inserted through the nose and pass through the stomach and into the small bowel beyond, thus ensuring that nutrition and hydration are delivered directly to the small bowel. These are also generally used in patients in whom the tube is placed as a short-term treatment.

- Gastrostomy tubes pass directly through the abdominal wall and into the stomach. Most gastroenterologists are trained to place gastrostomy tubes using endoscopic techniques. These gastrostomy tubes are referred to as PEG tubes (Figure 8-11). Gastrostomy tubes can remain in place for months or years.

- PEG-J tubes are PEG tubes with an internal extending tube that passes through the stomach and into

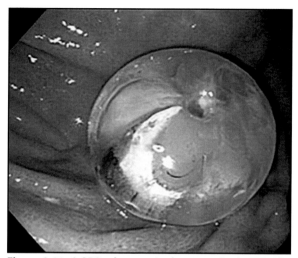

Figure 8-11. A PEG tube seen in the stomach via EGD. The water-filled balloon keeps the tube from falling out, and tube feeds are inserted into the stomach via the central lumen of the tube itself.

the small bowel and beyond in a patient who needs to be fed directly into the small bowel. The term refers to a PEG with a jejunal extension. These tubes can also remain in place for months or years.

- Percutaneous endoscopic jejunostomy tubes pass through the abdominal wall and directly into the small bowel (usually the jejunum) and completely bypass the esophagus and stomach. These tubes can also remain in place for months or years.

Once these tubes are placed, they need careful maintenance and monitoring, which are often performed by nurses. Patients with feeding tubes also need careful nutritional evaluation to determine the correct amount of calories and water they need in a given day.

TRANSLUMINAL PROCEDURES

Recent years have seen the rise of an entirely new field of endoscopic procedures, collectively referred to as *transluminal procedures*. The lumen of the gastrointestinal tract refers to the inside of the esophagus, stomach, or large and small intestines. Most endoscopic procedures traditionally take place within the lumen. Procedures like ERCP and EUS involve both intraluminal and extraluminal maneuvers but in very delicate and careful ways. Transluminal procedures, as the name implies, involve procedures that go through the wall of the esophagus, stomach, or bowel in a more florid way.

Since the inception of endoscopy, the mantra was "Don't perforate the bowel!" Transluminal procedures not only intentionally perforate the bowel, but also the endoscopist will often take steps to hold the perforation open, all so that the endoscope or other tools can traverse the perforation and enter another site to intervene on another structure or organ to help the patient.

The rise of transluminal procedures has been greatly facilitated by the invention of devices known as *LAMSs*. LAMSs hold open a perforation between 2 organs and allow endoscopes and other devices to go between the 2 bridged structures as needed (Figure 8-12). LAMSs are usually placed under EUS guidance.

The first transluminal procedure was the endoscopic drainage of pancreatic pseudocysts, wherein the endoscopist would intentionally perforate the stomach or bowel to access a pseudocyst and place stents between the cyst and the bowel to create a route for internal drainage, thus saving the patient from having to go to the operating room and having the cyst drained surgically.

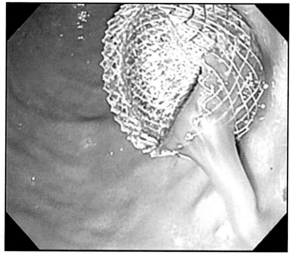

Figure 8-12. An endoscopic view of an LAMS draining a pseudocyst, showing how a transluminal gateway is held open. Note the drainage of pseudocyst fluid into the stomach.

Some examples of transluminal procedures include the following:

- **Endoscopic pseudocyst drainage:** This is the classic transluminal procedure. A pseudocyst that developed as a consequence of pancreatitis is connected to the stomach or bowel and allowed to drain internally, thus sparing the patient surgery.

- **Endoscopic drainage and debridement of walled-off pancreatic necrosis:** This is kind of the "big brother" of endoscopic pseudocyst drainage. Sometimes pancreatitis can be so bad that part (or all) of the pancreas dies. This dead tissue needs to be removed because it can often become infected or cause other problems if left in place. Using an LAMS, the stomach or small bowel can be perforated; the retroperitoneum, where the pancreas resides, can be accessed; and the dead tissue can be removed through the LAMS in pieces, thus saving the patient from undergoing surgery.

- **Endoscopic gallbladder drainage:** In general, if you have an inflamed or infected gallbladder, it should be removed surgically. Some patients with a sick gallbladder are too sick to undergo surgery. Historically, those patients had a tube placed into the gallbladder to drain the infection, but these tubes are often permanent and deeply unpopular with patients. Endoscopic gallbladder drainage, usually performed with an LAMS in an off-label manner, allows an artificial hole to be made between the gallbladder and the stomach or intestines so that the gallbladder can drain internally and the patient can avoid risky surgery or a drainage tube (Figure 8-13).

- **Endoscopic gastrojejunostomy:** Sometimes, often due to a tumor, the stomach or small bowel becomes obstructed, and patients cannot eat. Historically, these patients underwent a surgical bypass in which the small bowel was sewn to the stomach so food could get out. This procedure was called a *gastrojejunostomy*. Other options included putting a stent in the blocked bowel to open it up. Using an LAMS in an off-label manner, a gastrojejunostomy can be created endoscopically, thus avoiding surgery.

- **Endoscopic access to the stomach after gastric bypass:** When patients undergo a Roux-en-Y gastric bypass for weight loss, the stomach is no longer endoscopically accessible. Using an LAMS

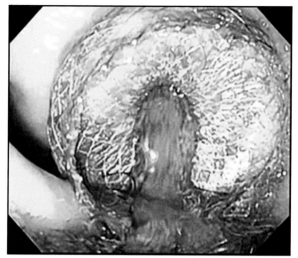

Figure 8-13. An endoscopic view of an LAMS used to drain the gallbladder in a nonsurgical candidate. Note the drainage of gallbladder sludge and bile to the stomach.

in an off-label manner, a conduit can be created between the gastric pouch and the stomach itself, allowing access to the stomach. This conduit can be used to perform ERCPs, gastric biopsies, and other procedures.

- **EUS-guided bile duct and pancreatic duct drainage:** Using EUS scopes and needles, a hole can be made between the bile ducts or the pancreatic ducts and the stomach or bowel. Stents can be placed across these sites to allow permanent drainage. These procedures are often performed when routine ERCP drainage of a blocked bile duct or pancreatic duct cannot be performed or has been tried and failed.

ADVANCED IMAGING

Endoscopy has gone far beyond a simple lighted tube that lets us see inside the gastrointestinal tract. Although most endoscopes use what is referred to as *white light*, the following special techniques exist that allow very high-resolution examinations to be performed:

- **Chromoendoscopy:** This technique involves the use of special dyes, either ingested by the patient or sprayed through the endoscope, that allow the lining of the gastrointestinal lumen to be seen in greatly enhanced detail. These are often very helpful when looking at polyps before removal or can be used to help find polyps in the first place, most commonly in patients with inflammatory bowel disease.

- **Optical coherence tomography (OCT):** OCT uses special probes to image the lining of the gastrointestinal tract in incredible detail, allowing structures as small as 8 microns (μm) to be seen. OCT is usually used to carefully inspect Barrett's esophagus for signs of precancerous change.

- **Confocal laser endomicroscopy:** Confocal laser endomicroscopy allows extreme magnification, even more than OCT, to the point where individual cells can be identified! OCT is often used to look for signs of precancerous change or cancer in the target tissue.

BIBLIOGRAPHY

Adler DG. Endoscopic gallbladder drainage. *Am J Gastroenterol.* 2019;114(5):700-702.

Adler DG, Cox K, Milliken M, et al. A large multicenter study analysis of adverse events associated with single operator cholangiopancreatoscopy. *Minerva Gastroenterol Dietol.* 2015;61(4):179-184.

Adler DG, Leighton JA, Davila RE, et al; ASGE. ASGE guideline: the role of endoscopy in acute non-variceal upper-GI hemorrhage [published correction appears in *Gastrointest Endosc.* 2005;61(2):356]. *Gastrointest Endosc.* 2004;60(4):497-504.

ASGE Standards of Practice Committee; Jain R, Maple JT, et al. The role of endoscopy in enteral feeding. *Gastrointest Endosc.* 2011;74(1):7-12.

ASGE Standards of Practice Committee; Maple JT, Ikenberry SO, et al. The role of endoscopy in the management of choledocholithiasis [published corrections appears in *Gastrointest Endosc.* 2012;75(1):230-230.e14]. *Gastrointest Endosc.* 2011;74(4):731-744.

Baxter NN, Goldwasser MA, Paszat LF, Saskin R, Urbach DR, Rabeneck L. Association of colonoscopy and death from colorectal cancer. *Ann Intern Med.* 2009;150(1):1-8.

Brenner H, Chang-Claude J, Seiler CM, Rickert A, Hoffmeister M. Protection from colorectal cancer after colonoscopy: a population-based, case-control study. *Ann Intern Med.* 2011;154(1):22-30.

Davila RE, Rajan E, Adler DG, et al; Standards of Practice Committee. ASGE guideline: the role of endoscopy in the patient with lower-GI bleeding. *Gastrointest Endosc.* 2005;62(5):656-660.

Elmunzer BJ, Scheiman JM, Lehman GA, et al; U.S. Cooperative for Outcomes Research in Endoscopy (USCORE). A randomized trial of rectal indomethacin to prevent post-ERCP pancreatitis. *N Engl J Med.* 2012;366(15):1414-1422.

Liu R, Cox Rn K, Siddiqui A, Feurer M, Baron T, Adler DG. Peroral cholangioscopy facilitates targeted tissue acquisition in patients with suspected cholangiocarcinoma. *Minerva Gastroenterol Dietol.* 2014;60(2):127-133.

Parbhu SK, Siddiqui AA, Murphy M, et al. Efficacy, safety, and outcomes of endoscopic retrograde cholangiopancreatography with per-oral pancreatoscopy: a multicenter experience. *J Clin Gastroenterol.* 2017;51(10):e101-e105.

Siddiqui AA, Adler DG, Nieto J, et al. EUS-guided drainage of peripancreatic fluid collections and necrosis by using a novel lumen-apposing stent: a large retrospective, multicenter U.S. experience (with videos). *Gastrointest Endosc.* 2016;83(4):699-707.

Trindade AJ, Benias PC, Kurupathi P, et al. Digital pancreatoscopy in the evaluation of main duct intraductal papillary mucinous neoplasm: a multicenter study. *Endoscopy.* 2018;50(11):1095-1098.

Index

acquired liver diseases, 142-148
    alcoholic liver disease, 142-144
    autoimmune hepatitis, 145-146
    Budd-Chiari syndrome, 147-148
    nonalcoholic fatty liver disease,
       144-145
       diagnosis of, 145
    primary biliary cholangitis,
       146-147
actively bleeding ulcers, 49
acute pancreatitis, 197-206
    causes, 199-201
    diagnosis, 201-202
    etiology, 199-201
    pathophysiology, 198
    treatment, 202-206
adenocarcinoma, pancreatic, 216-218
advanced imaging, 270
    chromoendoscopy, 270
    confocal laser endomicroscopy, 270
    optical coherence tomography, 270
alcoholic liver disease, 142-144
alpha-1 antitrypsin deficiency, 139-140
ampullary cancer, 189
ampullary diseases, 188-190
    ampullary adenomas, 188-189
anatomy, 71-75
anorectal disorders, 120-125
arteriovenous malformations, 95-96
ascites, cirrhosis, 132-134
autoimmune hepatitis, 145-146
AVMs. *See* Arteriovenous malformations

balloon enteroscopy, 248-250
Barrett's esophagus, 14-20
    diagnosis, 14-16

    long-segment, 16
    management, 17-20
       endoscopy, 19-20
       surgery, 18-19
    Prague classification, 17
    short-segment, 16
bile duct structures, 177-182
bile ducts, 161-192
bile leaks, 174-177
bile metabolism, 163-164
biliary colic, 167
biliary cysts, 187-188
Budd-Chiari syndrome, 147-148

cancer
    ampullary, 189
    colorectal, 114-119
    esophageal, 26-35
       clinical presentation, 28-30
       endoscopic treatments, 34-35
       endoscopic treatments
          for dysphagia in
          esophageal cancer,
          31-35
       esophagectomy, 30-31
       etiology, 27-28
       neoadjuvant therapy, 30-31
       pretreatment evaluation,
          28-30
       stents, 32-34
    gallbladder, 165, 179
    hepatocellular, 154-156
    metastatic, 181
    pancreatic, 177
    small bowel, 88-90
capsule endoscopy, 242-245

catabolism, liver, 130
celiac sprue, 75-78
cholangiocarcinoma, 165
cholangiography, 165
cholangiopancreatography, endoscopic
    retrograde, 253-258
cholangioscopy, 165
cholangitis, 165
    primary biliary, 146-147
cholecystectomy, 165
cholecystitis, 165, 167-170
choledochocele, 165
choledochoduodenostomy, 165
choledochojejunostomy, 165
choledocholithiasis, 165, 170-174
cholelithiasis, 165
chronic pancreatitis, 208-215
    etiology, 209-212
    symptoms, 212-214
    treatment, 214-215
cirrhosis, 131-137
    ascites, 132-134
    bleeding, 134-135
    hepatic encephalopathy, 135-137
clean-based ulcers, 48
colitis, 103-112
    collagenous, 111-112
colon, 99-119
    anatomy, 100-102
    cancer, 114-119
    colitis, 103-112
    collagenous colitis, 111-112
    colonic surgery terminology,
        102-103
    colorectal cancer, 114-119
    diagram of, 101
    diverticulitis, 112-114
    diverticulosis, 112-114
    function, 100
    infectious colitis, 109-110
    ischemic colitis, 110-111
    lymphocytic colitis, 111-112
    microscopic colitis, 111-112
    ulcerative colitis, 103-109
colonic surgery, terminology, 102-103
colonoscope, 246-247
colonoscopy, 233-242
    diagnostic colonoscopy, 235-237
    polyp detection tools, 239-242
    polypectomy, 238-239
    screening colonoscopy, 234-235
    surveillance colonoscopy, 235

    therapeutic colonoscopy, 237-238
    types, 234-242
colorectal cancer, 114-119
confocal laser endomicroscopy, 270
Crohn's disease, 78-86
    antibiotics, 83
    biologics, 84-85
    biosimilars, 85
        aminosalicylates, 85-86
    corticosteroids, 82
    medications, 82-86
    nonsteriodal immunosuppressive
        drugs, 83-84
cystic lesions, 220-223
    intraductal papillary mucinous
        neoplasms, 221
    mucinous cystadenomas, 221
    serous cystadenomas, 221
    solid pseudopapillary tumors, 221

detoxification/catabolism, liver, 130
    storage, 131
diagnostic colonoscopy, 235-237
diarrhea of small bowel origin, 90-95
    functional disorders, 93-94
    infections, 90-91
    inflammatory diarrhea, 93
    mechanisms, 90-94
    motility disorders, 92
    osmotic diarrhea, 92-93
    secretory diarrhea, 91
    short bowel syndrome, 91-92
    side effects, medication, 94-95
diculafoy lesion, 49
Dieulafoy lesion, 97
diverticulitis, 112-114
diverticulosis, 112-114
drug-induced bile duct disease, 186
duplication cysts, 63-64
dysphagia, 3-7
    achalasia, 4-5
    eosinophilic esophagitis, 5-6

end-stage liver disease scores, 157-158
endoscopic retrograde
    cholangiopancreatography,
    250-260
    accessories, 253-258
    balloons, 254
    baskets, 254
    brushes, 255
    cannulas, 253

cholangioscopes, 255-258
guidewires, 253
indications, 258-260
pancreatoscopes, 255-258
sphincterotomes, 253-254
stents, 254-255
endoscopic therapy, 49-53
hemostatic powders, 52-53
injection therapy, 50
mechanical therapy, 50-52
thermal therapy, 50
endoscopic ultrasound, 260-263
endoscopy, 225-272
advanced imaging, 270
chromoendoscopy, 270
confocal laser
endomicroscopy, 270
optical coherence tomography,
270
capsule endoscopy, 242-245
colonoscopy, 233-242
diagnostic colonoscopy,
235-237
polyp detection tools,
239-242
polypectomy, 238-239
screening colonoscopy,
234-235
surveillance colonoscopy,
235
therapeutic colonoscopy,
237-238
types, 234-242
endoscopic retrograde
cholangiopancreatography,
250-260
accessories, 253-258
balloons, 254
baskets, 254
brushes, 255
cannulas, 253
cholangioscopes, 255-258
guidewires, 253
indications, 258-260
pancreatoscopes, 255-258
sphincterotomes, 253-254
stents, 254-255
endoscopic ultrasound, 260-263
enteroscopy, 246-250
balloon enteroscopy, 248-250
colonoscope, 246-247
push enteroscope, 247-248

esophagogastroduodenoscopy,
228-232
diagnostic upper endoscopy,
229-230
standard upper endoscope,
228-229
therapeutic upper
endoscope, 229
therapeutic upper
endoscopy, 230-232
feeding tubes, 264-265
gastrostomy tubes, 264
nasoenteric tubes, 264
nasogastric tubes, 264
PEG-J tubes, 264-265
percutaneous endoscopic
jejunostomy tubes,
265
informed consent, 227-228
sedation, 227
team, 226
transluminal procedures, 266-269
endoscopic access after
gastric bypass,
268-269
endoscopic gallbladder
drainage, 268
endoscopic
gastrojejunostomy,
268
endoscopic pseudocyst
drainage, 267
EUS-guided bile duct/
pancreatic duct
drainage, 269
walled-off pancreatic
necrosis, endoscopic
drainage/
debridement, 267-268
enteroscopy, 246-250
balloon enteroscopy, 248-250
colonoscope, 246-247
push enteroscope, 247-248
erosion ulcers, 47-48
esophageal cancer, 26-35
clinical presentation, 28-30
endoscopic treatments, 31-35
stents, 32-34
esophagectomy, 30-31
etiology, 27-28
neoadjuvant therapy, 30-31
pretreatment evaluation, 28-30

esophageal varices, 21-26
  endoscopic evaluation, 22-23
  endoscopic therapy, 23-26
    baloons, 26
    band ligation, 24-25
    sclerotherapy, 25-26
    shunts, 26
  pathophysiology, 21-22
  primary prevention of esophageal
    variceal bleeding using
    medications, 23
esophagogastroduodenoscopy, 228-232
  diagnostic upper endoscopy,
    229-230
  standard upper endoscope,
    228-229
  therapeutic upper endoscope, 229
  therapeutic upper endoscopy,
    230-232
esophagus, 1-36
  anatomy, 1-3
  Barrett's esophagus, 14-20
    diagnosis, 14-16
    endoscopy, 19-20
    long-segment, 16
    management, 17-20
    Prague classification, 17
    short-segment, 16
    surgery, 18-19
  cancer, 26-35
    clinical presentation, 28-30
    endoscopic treatments,
      34-35
    endoscopic treatments
      for dysphagia in
      esophageal cancer,
      31-35
    esophagectomy, 30-31
    etiology, 27-28
    neoadjuvant therapy, 30-31
    pretreatment evaluation,
      28-30
    stents, 32-34
    subsequent esophagectomy,
      30-31
  dysphagia, 3-7
    achalasia, 4-5
    eosinophilic esophagitis, 5-6
esophageal cancer, 26-35
  clinical presentation, 28-30
  endoscopic treatments
    for dysphagia in

    esophageal cancer,
      31-35
  esophagectomy, 30-31
  etiology, 27-28
  neoadjuvant therapy, 30-31
  pretreatment evaluation,
    28-30
  stents, 32-34
esophageal varices, 21-26
  balloons, 26
  band ligation, 24-25
  endoscopic evaluation,
    22-23
  endoscopic therapy, 23-26
  pathophysiology, 21-22
  primary prevention of
    esophageal variceal
    bleeding using
    medications, 23
  sclerotherapy, 25-26
  shunts, 26
gastroesophageal reflux disease, 7-14
  antacids, 12
  diagnosis, 9-11
  H2 receptor antagonists, 12
  medical treatment, 11-12
  pathophysiology, 7-9
  proton pump inhibitors,
    13-14
  physiology, 1-3
EUS-guided bile duct/pancreatic duct
  drainage, 269

feeding, 264-265
feeding tubes, 264-265
  gastrostomy tubes, 264
  nasoenteric tubes, 264
  nasogastric tubes, 264
  PEG-J tubes, 264-265
  percutaneous endoscopic
    jejunostomy tubes, 265
functions of liver, 129-131
  catabolism, 130
  detoxification/catabolism, 130
  storage, 131
  synthetic functions, 130

gallbladder, 161-192
gallstones, 166
gastric acid production, 39-41
gastric antral vascular ectasia, 64-65
gastric motility, 65-70

gastric tumors, 53-64
  duplication cysts, 63-64
  leiomyomas, 61-63
  stromal tumors, gastrointestinal, 59-61
  tumors of mucosal origin, 54-56
    mucosa-associated lymphoid tissue, 56
  tumors of submucosal origin, 56-64
    duplication cysts, 63-64
    extrinsic compression from another organ, 64
    gastrointestinal stromal tumors, 59-61
    leiomyomas, 61-63
gastroesophageal reflux disease, 7-14
  antacids, 12
  diagnosis, 9-11
  H2 receptor antagonists, 12
  medical treatment, 11-12
  pathophysiology, 7-9
  proton pump inhibitors, 13-14
gastrostomy tubes, 264
GAVE. *See* Gastric antral vascular ectasia

Helicobacter pylori, peptic ulcer disease, 46
hemochromatosis, hereditary, 138-139
hemostatic powders, 52-53
hemosuccus pancreaticus, 97
hepatic encephalopathy, 135-137
hepaticojejunostomy, 165
hepatitis, autoimmune, 145-146
hepatitis A virus, 149-150
hepatitis B virus, 150-151
hepatitis C virus, 151-153
  treatment, 152-153
hepatitis D virus, 153
hepatitis E virus, 154
hepatocellular cancer, 154-156
hereditary liver diseases, 137-142
  alpha-1 antitrypsin deficiency, 139-140
  hereditary hemochromatosis, 138-139
  hereditary hyperbilirubinemia, 141-142
  Wilson's disease, 140-141
hiatal hernias, 42-44
  risk factors, 43
  treatment, 44
HIV cholangiopathy, 185-186
hyperbilirubinemia, hereditary, 141-142

immunoglobulin subclass 4-associated cholangiopathy, 186
infectious colitis, 109-110
inflammatory diarrhea, 93
informed consent, 227-228
injection therapy, 50
intraductal papillary mucinous neoplasms, 221
ischemic colitis, 110-111

jejunostomy tubes, percutaneous endoscopic, 265

Kaposi's sarcoma, 97

leiomyomas, 61-63
liver, 127-160
  acquired liver diseases, 142-148
    alcoholic liver disease, 142-144
    autoimmune hepatitis, 145-146
    Budd-Chiari syndrome, 147-148
    nonalcoholic fatty liver disease, 144-145
    primary biliary cholangitis, 146-147
  anatomy, 128-129
  biliary anatomy, 128-129
  cirrhosis, 131-137
    ascites, 132-134
    bleeding, 134-135
    hepatic encephalopathy, 135-137
  functions, 129-131
    catabolism, 130
    detoxification/catabolism, 130-131
    synthetic functions, 130
  hepatocellular cancer, 154-156
  hereditary liver diseases, 137-142
    alpha-1 antitrypsin deficiency, 139-140
    hereditary hemochromatosis, 138-139
    hereditary hyperbilirubinemia, 141-142
    Wilson's disease, 140-141
  liver transplantation, 156-160

end-stage liver disease
                scores, 157-158
        life after, 159-160
        recipients, 157
        surgical options, 158-159
    microscopic anatomy, 129
    vascular anatomy, 128
    viral hepatitis, 148-154
        hepatitis A virus, 149-150
        hepatitis B virus, 150-151
        hepatitis C virus, 151-153
        hepatitis D virus, 153
        hepatitis E virus, 154
long-segment Barrett's esophagus, 16
lymphocytic colitis, 111-112

mechanical therapy, 50-52
Meckel's diverticulum, 96-97
metastatic cancer, 181
microscopic colitis, 111-112
mild pancreatitis, 202-203
mucinous cystadenomas, 221

nasoenteric tubes, 264
nasogastric tubes, 264
neuroendocrine tumors, 218-220
nonalcoholic fatty liver disease, 144-145
    diagnosis of, 145

optical coherence tomography, 270
osmotic diarrhea, 92-93

pancreas, 193-224
    acute pancreatitis, 197-206
        causes, 199-201
        diagnosis, 201-202
        etiology, 199-201
        pathophysiology, 198
        treatment, 202-206
    anatomy, 194-197
    chronic pancreatitis, 208-215
        etiology, 209-212
        symptoms, 212-214
        treatment, 214-215
    cystic lesions, 220-223
        intraductal papillary
                mucinous
                neoplasms, 221
        mucinous cystadenomas,
                221
        serous cystadenomas, 221

        solid pseudopapillary
                tumors, 221
    imaging studies, 206-208
        computed tomography
                scans, 207
        endoscopic ultrasound, 208
        magnetic resonance
                imaging scans, 208
        right upper quadrant
                transabdominal
                ultrasound, 207
        standard x-rays, 206
    mild pancreatitis, 202-203
    physiology, 194-197
    severe pancreatitis, 203-206
    solid pancreatic tumors, 216-220
        neuroendocrine tumors,
                218-220
        pancreatic adenocarcinoma,
                216-218
pancreatic cancer, 177
pancreatic tumors, solid, 216-220
        neuroendocrine tumors, 218-220
        pancreatic adenocarcinoma,
                216-218
PEG-J tubes, 264-265
peptic ulcer disease, 45-53
        Helicobacter pylori, 46
        hypersecretory states, 47
        nonsteroidal anti-inflammatory
                drugs, 45
        stress ulcers, 46
        types of endoscopic therapy, 49-53
                hemostatic powders, 52-53
                injection therapy, 50
                mechanical therapy, 50-52
                thermal therapy, 50
        types of ulcers, 47-49
                actively bleeding ulcers, 49
                clean-based ulcers, 48
                diculafoy lesion, 49
                erosions, 47-48
                ulcers with flat pigmented
                        spots, 48-49
                ulcers with nonbleeding
                        visible vessel, 49
                ulcers with overlying, 49
percutaneous endoscopic jejunostomy
        tubes, 265
physiology, 71-75
polyp detection tools, 239-242
polypectomy, 238-239

Prague classification, Barrett's esophagus, 17
primary biliary cholangitis, 146-147
primary sclerosing cholangitis, 182-185
pseudopapillary tumors, solid, 221
push enteroscope, 247-248

rectum, 120-125
    anorectal disorders, 120-125

SBO. *See* Small intestine bacterial overgrowth
secretory diarrhea, 91
serous cystadenomas, 221
severe pancreatitis, 203-206
short bowel syndrome, 91-92
small bowel bleeding, 95-97
    arteriovenous malformations, 95-96
    causes, 95-97
    Dieulafoy lesion, 97
    hemosuccus pancreaticus, 97
    Kaposi's sarcoma, 97
    Meckel's diverticulum, 96-97
    polyps, 96
    tumors, 96
    ulcers, 96
small bowel cancer, 88-90
small intestine, 71-98
    anatomy, 71-75
    celiac sprue, 75-78
    Crohn's disease, 78-86
        aminosalicylates, 85-86
        antibiotics, 83
        biologics, 84-85
        biosimilars, 85
        corticosteroids, 82
        medications, 82-86
        nonsteriodal immunosuppressive drugs, 83-84
    diarrhea of small bowel origin, 90-95
        functional disorders producing diarrhea, 93-94
        infections, 90-91
        inflammatory diarrhea, 93
        mechanisms, 90-94
        medication side effects, 94-95
        motility disorders, 92
        osmotic diarrhea, 92-93
        secretory diarrhea, 91

    short bowel syndrome, 91-92
    diseases, 75-97
    physiology, 71-75
    small bowel bleeding, 95-97
        arteriovenous malformations, 95-96
        causes, 95-97
        Dieulafoy lesion, 97
        hemosuccus pancreaticus, 97
        Kaposi's sarcoma, 97
        Meckel's diverticulum, 96-97
        polyps, 96
        tumors, 96
        ulcers, 96
    small bowel cancer, 88-90
small intestine bacterial overgrowth, 86-88
solid pancreatic tumors, 216-220
    neuroendocrine tumors, 218-220
    pancreatic adenocarcinoma, 216-218
solid pseudopapillary tumors, 221
stomach, 37-70
    anatomy, 38-39
    gastric acid production, 39-41
    gastric antral vascular ectasia, 64-65
    gastric motility, 65-70
    gastric tumors, 53-64
        tumors of mucosal origin, 54-56
        tumors of submucosal origin, 56-64
    hiatal hernias, 42-44
        risk factors, 43
        treatment, 44
    peptic ulcer disease, 45-53
        Helicobacter pylori, 46
        hypersecretory states, 47
        nonsteroidal anti-inflammatory drugs, 45
        stress ulcers, 46
        types of endoscopic therapy, 49-53
        types of ulcers, 47-49
    vitamin B12, 41-42
stress ulcers, 46
stromal tumors, gastrointestinal, 59-61

surveillance colonoscopy, 235
synthetic functions, liver, 130

team, endoscopy, 226
therapeutic colonoscopy, 237-238
thermal therapy, 50
transluminal procedures, 266-269
    endoscopic access after gastric
        bypass, 268-269
    endoscopic gallbladder drainage,
        268
    endoscopic gastrojejunostomy, 268
    endoscopic pseudocyst drainage,
        267
    EUS-guided bile duct/pancreatic
        duct drainage, 269
    walled-off pancreatic necrosis,
        endoscopic drainage/
        debridement, 267-268
transplantation, liver, 156-160
    end-stage liver disease scores,
        157-158
    life after, 159-160
    recipients, 157
    surgical options, 158-159
tubes, feeding, 264-265
    gastrostomy tubes, 264
    nasoenteric tubes, 264
    nasogastric tubes, 264
    PEG-J tubes, 264-265
    percutaneous endoscopic
        jejunostomy tubes, 265

UC. *See* Ulcerative colitis
ulcer types, 47-49
    actively bleeding ulcers, 49
    clean-based ulcers, 48

diculafoy lesion, 49
    erosions, 47-48
    ulcers with flat pigmented spots,
        48-49
    ulcers with nonbleeding visible
        vessel, 49
    ulcers with overlying, 49
ulcerative colitis, 103-109
ulcers with flat pigmented spots, 48-49
ulcers with nonbleeding visible vessel, 49
ulcers with overlying, 49

varices, esophageal, 21-26
    endoscopic evaluation, 22-23
    endoscopic therapy, 23-26
        band ligation, 24-25
        sclerotherapy, 25-26
        shunts, 26
    pathophysiology, 21-22
    primary prevention of esophageal
        variceal bleeding using
        medications, 23
viral hepatitis, 148-154
    hepatitis A virus, 149-150
    hepatitis B virus, 150-151
    hepatitis C virus, 151-153
    hepatitis D virus, 153
    hepatitis E virus, 154
vitamin B12, 41-42

walled-off pancreatic necrosis, endoscopic
    drainage/debridement, 267-268
Wilson's disease, 140-141

Printed in the United States
by Baker & Taylor Publisher Services